Professionalism in Nursing
A Foundation for Practice

Revised First Edition

Maria A. Revell

Middle Tennessee State University

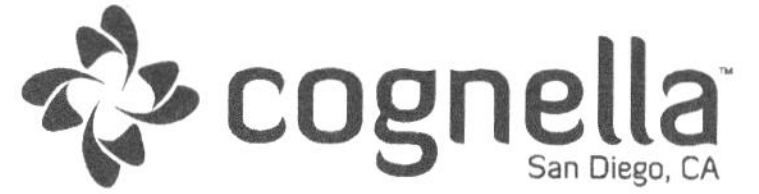

cognella

San Diego, CA

Bassim Hamadeh, CEO and Publisher
Christopher Foster, General Vice President
Michael Simpson, Vice President of Acquisitions
Jessica Knott, Managing Editor
Kevin Fahey, Cognella Marketing Manager
Jess Busch, Senior Graphic Designer
Zina Craft, Acquisitions Editor
Jamie Giganti, Senior Project Editor
Brian Fahey, Licensing Associate

First published in the United States of America in 2013 by Cognella, Inc.

Printed in the United States of America

ISBN: 978-1-62131-551-3 (pbk) / 978-1-62131-552-0 (br)

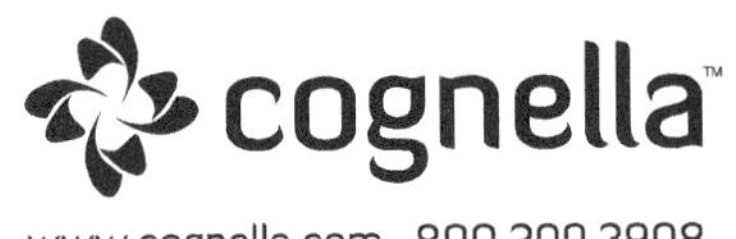
www.cognella.com 800.200.3908

Contents

Preface

The pace of change is relentless. This pace will continue into the future with society requiring the need for the services of nurses more than ever. The nursing profession is under tremendous challenges to respond to these societal health related changes. As society changes so will the structure that supports health care. Professional nurses will have challenges to patient care based on many changes in these health care systems. These challenges create increased responsibilities for nurses in the delivery of direct care activities. These activities will not only include care in numerous settings but also require a focus on preventive and chronic care. These activities will require that the nurse engage in focused patient education inclusive of culture and address other behaviors that promote self-care management.

It is imperative that as professional nurses we develop attitudes that actively reflect critical thinking and clinical wisdom. This thinking and wisdom is grown through engagement in activities that promote appropriate ethical and legal decisions in patient care management. These forms of thinking should be mixed with nursing theories and models that endorse evidence based interventions. This first edition is designed to give individuals who use the book a candle to light or rekindle their passion for nursing. It will not only give you an entering perspective of the professional nurse but a look at what nursing is and can be.

Chapter 1: Nursing's History

The Road Traveled

By Marcia A. Pugh, DNP, MBA, HCM, RN

Nursing care was provided by individuals in society long before nursing was identified as an occupation and subsequent profession. In medieval times, men provided care for the ill as part of their daily-life activities. During the Victorian era, care was provided by women paupers from workhouses. Women were the primary care providers for the injured and ill in the early Americas. In 1873 formal teaching and learning was implemented based on the British model of education. There was no conceptual base for nursing education, so foundationally this education was managed by administrators and medical entities. Nursing has evolved through the centuries to focus on evidence that supports its specific patient care activities. This chapter will take you through nursing's evolution and introduce you to key individuals in its progression from occupation to profession.

Before nurses evolved to establish a formal structure for helping the sick, illness and suffering were a part of everyday life. Since the beginning of time, there have been afflictions and illnesses. Those with the misfortune to experience such were cared for by family. With the nuclear and extended family all under the same roof, there was no lack of available hands. This, however, did not guarantee health. With thatched roof houses, water from any source available, lack of indoor plumbing and refrigeration, and all manner of insects and animals ever-present in the home, illness was a norm. Treatment sometimes meant a concoction of herbs and animal entrails. Caring for the sick only meant palliative care until the person succumbed to their illness or "miraculously" returned to health.

A History of Tending the Sick

The nursing profession is linked to Florence Nightingale. But long before Nightingale, there were people who tended the sick. During the Crusades, those who cared for the wounded and ill were called Hospitallers. These individuals performed this work not only out of duty, but out of personal preference. During the Middle Ages, nursing care activities were provided by male-dominated religious, military, and secular orders. The Knights of Saint John was one such religious order who performed these activities. One predominant principle of this order was devotion to duty in care for the sick. This became a standard in nursing across the ages and continues to be a standard in nursing today.

Many Catholic orders cared for the sick in the Middle Ages. These individuals cared for the sick with information passed down from person to person through apprenticeships. These caring and humane activities lacked hygienic measures and were administered under primitive conditions. Institutional primordial provisions, coupled with overcrowding, also made it necessary to go into the communities to care for the sick.

During the Reformation, Catholic support for the monasteries and institutions designed to care for the sick severely waned, thus allowing abolition by the Protestants. Many Catholic hospitals of the time were replaced by workhouses and almshouses. These were aimed primarily at the poor and destitute. Care in these new institutions was provided by pardoned criminals, alcoholics, and aged prostitutes. Nurses in these times were depicted by Charles Dickens in the portrayal of his character, Sairey Gamp. This "nurse" was more concerned with her own comforts than those of her patients. This was an attitude distinctly different from prior care providers.

The Reformation brought a new wave of thinkers and philosophers. These individuals began to view values and ideals from a different perspective. The evolution of nursing took on a new dimension with the onset of the Industrial Revolution, when capitalism, individualism, and freedom of thought formed the foundation for a more democratic view of government. This view took several years to evolve an accepting attitude, where women worked outside the home. It was also unthinkable that women from upstanding families worked to tend the sick and dying. This was the era in which Florence Nightingale was born.

Florence Nightingale

Florence Nightingale was the second daughter born to an upstanding aristocratic family in Victorian England in 1820. She had a carefree life and was well educated in languages (Latin, German, French, and Greek), mathematics, science, and politics, to name a few. These laid the foundation for her future innovations in nursing.

While Nightingale was young, she often visited the sick as part of her aristocratic custom. This work suited her and gave her a sense of purpose. When Nightingale was 30 years old (Figure 2-2), she entered a training program for nurses in Kaiserworth, Germany. This three-year training program preceded her continued training in Paris under the Sisters of Charity. By the age of 33, Nightingale had become superintendent of an "Establishment for gentle women during illness."

The Crimean War paved the way for Nightingale to exhibit her exceptional administrative and organizational abilities learned as a child. Responding to an appeal by the minister of war, Nightingale and several nurses went to care for British soldiers injured in the war effort. When she arrived at the Scutari Barracks Hospital, the conditions were unbelievably horrible. The 1500-patient facility had soldiers crowded into dirty, poorly ventilated wards. The area was filled with filth and vermin. Poorly

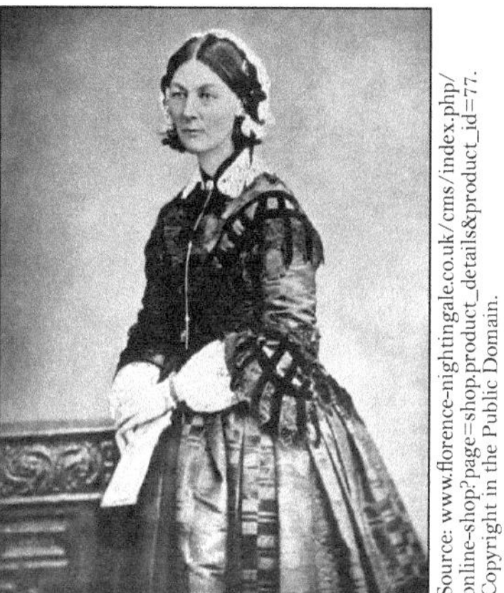

Figure 1. Florence Nightingale (1820–1910).

cooked food was served to the sick and injured at irregularly long intervals. Soldiers were covered with dirt and some lay on straw floor mats. Many were still in their uniforms stained with their own blood. Death in this facility occurred not related to battlefield injuries, but rather by cholera and disease.

Upon seeing these horrible conditions, Nightingale set about making life better for these sick and wounded soldiers. Despite military officer opposition, she achieved order in the health care facilities. She established care based on cleanliness requirements for patients and their surroundings, and managed to achieve total reorganization of these facilities. This development resulted from statistical information she retrieved and analyzed. She kept detailed data on Scutari soldier morbidity and mortality during the Crimean War. Nightingale monitored and gathered data through nightly rounds in the dark halls and rooms of soldiers in the facility, and was thus known as "Lady with the Lamp." These analyses served to change not only military perspectives, but those of society regarding care of the sick. These analyses resulted in the idea that sick and wounded soldiers had the right to adequate nutrition, suitable living quarters, and appropriate health care. These interventions, built on evidence-based results, achieved a significant reduction of mortality from 43% to 2% in the Crimean War. Nightingale definitely established a correlation between environmental conditions and health status (Johnson & Webber, 2009).

From the war years, Nightingale moved toward working to improve the education of nurses. In 1860 the Nightingale School and Home for Nurses was established at St. Thomas' Hospital, which improved public perception and promoted discipline in nursing. Due to illness, she was not able to take an administrative position in the school. Despite this, she was involved and offered advice based on her Crimean War experience. In 1860 she published *Notes on Nursing: What It Is and What It Is Not.* In this document, she called nursing an art that encompassed activities that promoted good health and healing activities. Nightingale stated that education was imperative to promoting the nursing profession. Nightingale was a proficient writer and author during her lifetime. She was the keystone for mastering a body of knowledge specific to nursing.

The Influence of War on Nursing in America
Women of War Who Nursed the Sick

War has been an important impetus for nursing. Just as it was foundational to nursing in England, war served to promote nursing in America. The Civil War served as the stimulus for nursing's foundation in America. During the Civil War, there were many wounded on both sides of the fighting. Union and Confederate soldiers suffered as a result of poor sanitation and improper nutrition and care activities. Approximately 2,000 women served as volunteer nurses in North and South military hospitals during the American Civil War. These women served under some of the most horrific circumstances and rendered aid to mutilated and dying men. These women served with little recognition for the work they did in helping men to recovery or death.

Hannah Anderson Ropes (1809–1863)

Hannah Anderson Ropes was born in New Gloucester, Maine, in 1809 to a prominent attorney family. Her personal convictions were developed in childhood. She was strongly opposed to slavery. During the prewar era, she gained recognition as a reformer and abolitionist. It was only after the loss of her husband's support (he moved and left the family) and she was left to raise two small children that she became increasingly active in the abolitionist movement and westward expansion. Ropes nursed sick family and friends, as many women did during that time. It was at this time in her life that she was deeply affected by a copy of Nightingale's *Notes on Nursing* given to her by a family member. As a result, she volunteered to serve as a nurse when her son served in the Civil War. In 1862 Ropes worked in a Union hospital. Conditions were appalling and extended beyond a lack of sanitation, but also included cruel treatment by those in charge of the care for these soldiers. She worked to provide good food, a clean environment, and displayed a true sense of caring for the wounded. When Ropes witnessed soldier mistreatment by those in charge of providing their care (the steward and chief surgeon), she reported these behaviors directly to the secretary of war, which resulted in an official inspection of the conditions at the facility and the arrest of these two individuals, resulting in a change of administrators. Her efforts brought about remarkable changes for a woman in a male-dominated military environment. She was soon made head matron of the Union Hotel Hospital in Georgetown, a neighborhood outside Washington, D.C. With her prior contacts secured in her roles of reformer and abolitionist, Ropes was able to secure supplies and care necessities for wounded soldiers. This allowed her to put sanitation components pioneered by Nightingale in place. She worked to put her beliefs related to healthy surroundings, good food, and humanitarian treatment into nursing practice. Her concerns over the brutally indifferent treatment of soldiers caused her to ruthlessly battle the system on their behalf. Like so many of the soldiers she cared for, she succumbed to typhoid pneumonia at the age of 54.

Dorothea Lynde Dix (1802–1887)

Dorothea Lynde Dix was a champion for the mentally ill and those in prisons. She initiated her work in Massachusetts after observing their ill treatment and extremely poor conditions. This was her life's work for more than 20 years. During this time, she campaigned from state to state, addressing state legislators to effect positive change. Dix went from institution to institution, systematically observing and documenting her findings. She was so successful in her ability to initiate change that she was appointed superintendent of the female nurses of the Army by the secretary of war. Although she had no formal nurse's training, she was able to recruit more than 2,000 women to serve in the Union Army during the Civil War (American Nurses' Association, 2011). In this position, Dix was in charge of all female nurses working in the army hospitals. She served in this position throughout the entire war period without compensation for any of this work. Her recruitment efforts of other women worked to verify that women could work effectively in these settings. She was the first to implement a dress code in order to give female nurses more credibility among the ranks of the military men. Dix labored to improve the welfare of nurses and patients alike, recruiting not only female nurses, but often soliciting resources from private sources when these were not supplied by the government. Following completion of her duty in the military, she returned to continue working with the mentally ill and promote a better lifestyle for these individuals.

Susie King Taylor (1848–1912)

Susie King Taylor was born a slave in the state of Georgia. She had a very different experience as a child and was a slave of the Grest family. Despite her slave status, she was treated affectionately by the plantation owner's wife, who set the standard for how King judged potential relationships between blacks and whites. As a slave, she was not allowed to obtain an education. It was only after she visited her freed grandmother that her education began. During the war efforts, the family was moved in an attempt to secure safety. It was at this time that she met and married her husband. When she was living in Port Royal Island, off the South Carolina coast, her husband joined an all-black unit and she moved with him as the unit moved about the area fighting. She served as nurse and caretaker, also teaching many men to read and write during this time. In 1863 King began to nurse the wounded as they returned, battle-weary and injured. She worked with Clara Barton when caring for black soldiers in South Carolina. She volunteered for over three years in this capacity, despite the fact that she had no formal medical training. After the war ended in 1865, she focused her teaching efforts on children. She worked in education until the 1870s, at which time she remarried and continued her nursing efforts by joining and later becoming president of the Women's Relief Corps. King worked for the organization until her death.

Mary Ann Bickerdyke (1817–1901)

Mary Ann Bickerdyke had a relatively uneventful lifestyle until age 43. After the loss of an infant daughter, she started reading books on medicine in an effort to learn about health. In a sermon, she heard how Union soldiers received poor medical care, and was determined to work and improve this situation. She initiated a drive to collect medical supplies in her hometown and personally delivered these to the nearest Union base in Illinois. Upon seeing the terrible conditions of the camp's medical clinic, Bickerdyke stayed and started washing bedding and clothes, cooking, and cleaning soldier's wounds. She enlisted a small group of volunteer women to help her continue this work. She later moved from the hospital to the frontline, where she insisted in working alongside the medical staff. For her work, she was hired in an official capacity by the U.S. Sanitary Commission until it was disbanded at the war's conclusion. After that ended, Bickerdyke continued to work with recuperating soldiers. Her work extended to promoting services for Union veterans. She worked to get compensation that had been earned but never paid along with pensions. For her work with the Union army, she is remembered as "Mother to the Boys in Blue."

Clara Barton (1821–1912)

Clarissa Harlowe Barton, or Clara, she wished to be called, did not start out to work with the sick. This evolved as a result of an initiative she began in Massachusetts. While working in the U.S. Patent Office, she witnessed soldiers returning from war. As new recruits, these returning soldiers often had nothing more than the clothes on their backs. Their disheveled appearances and poor medical care on the battlefield meant some were disfigured, and their appearance confused and frightened the townspeople. Barton recognized that something needed to be done and organized a relief effort for these men. Her independent campaign carried her into the battlefield, where she set up a makeshift hospital to care for sick and dying soldiers. From this work, she became known as the "Angel of the Battlefield." With the success of her soldier relief efforts, she was granted permission to travel with army ambulances to comfort the sick and wounded while nursing them. Barton continued this work for three years, becoming nationally known for her caring work with casualties from the Battle of the Wilderness and Bermuda Hundred. During this time, she would write families to inform them of their soldier in the field. Her work behind the lines prompted an appointment by President Lincoln to locate men listed as missing, and when information was obtained, to notify families of the disposition of their loved ones. She established the Office of Correspondence with Friends of the Missing Men of the United States Army, which she operated for four years. Barton was instrumental in answering over 63,000 letters and identifying over 22,000 missing men (American Red Cross, n.d.). Today, this has become a valuable service of the Red Cross. In 1881 this work culminated in the establishment of the Red Cross. This organization was the fruit of all the efforts she made over her lifetime. Barton worked with the Red Cross until her resignation in 1904.

Other Women in U.S. Nursing

Linda Anne Judson Richards (1841–1930)

Linda Richards began her career as a schoolteacher, and after ten years began working as a nurse at Boston Hospital in 1870. In 1872 she began training at the New England Hospital for Women and Children and was the program's first graduate. This program was run by female physicians who based their one-year program on Florence Nightingale's principles. After graduation, she worked as night-shift supervisor at Bellevue Hospital in New York. In 1874 she returned to Boston, and was named superintendent of the Boston Training School. Through astute managerial skills, she was able to increase respect for the program, as it now was recognized as one of the best programs in the country. Richards traveled to England to work in an intensive nursing program of study. She studied at St. Thomas' Hospital in London. She was able to work with Nightingale, who recommended that she continue her studies at King's College Hospital and the Edinburgh Royal Infirmary in Scotland. Upon Richards's return to the states in 1878, she used her learned skills and expertise to assist in the organization of the Boston City Hospital training program. She was subsequently named matron of the hospital and superintendent of the school. Richards worked in these positions until 1885. Later in this same year, she traveled to Japan to establish the first nurse training program in that country. She remained in Japan for five years to supervise the school at Doshisha Hospital Kyoto. She subsequently returned to the United States. She worked in nursing for an additional 20 years. During this time, Richards established and directed nurse-training programs in Philadelphia, Massachusetts, and Michigan. Through her efforts, nursing programs progressed to an international level.

Mary Eliza Mahoney (1845–1926)

Mary Eliza Mahoney was the first African American registered nurse in the United States. Her interest in nursing started in her teen years as a free individual (not born into slavery). She worked for 15 years performing domestic duties and serving as an unofficial nurse's assistant at the New England Hospital for Women and Children in Massachusetts. At the age of 33, she made a conscious decision to enroll in a very difficult nursing program of the time. Nursing classes were challenging and programs were rigorous. In her class of approximately 40 students, only four completed the program—Mahoney was the only African American. Following graduation, she registered with the Nurses Directory in Boston and worked primarily as a private duty nurse. During her 30 professional years, she worked in states along the Eastern Seaboard of the United States. and ended her maiden (never married) nursing career working for 10 years as director of the Howard Orphan Asylum for Black Children in New York. In 1896 Mahoney was one of the original members of the predominantly white Nurses Associated Alumnae of the United States organization, which later became known as the American Nurses Association. She was cofounder of the National Association of Colored Graduate Nurses in 1908, which was later dissolved.

Isabel Adams Hampton Robb (1860–1910)

Isabel Hampton Robb received her training at the Bellevue Hospital Training School. Upon her graduation in 1883, she moved to Rome and worked at St. Paul's House, a small hospital for English and American travelers. Following this time, she returned to the United States and was appointed superintendent of nurses at the Illinois Training School for Nurses at Chicago's Cook County Hospital. In this post she was very instrumental in changing the training curricula for nurses. She abolished the practice of private duty nursing as a clinical experience. She affiliated with other hospitals to broaden the nurses' experience and developed the first grading policy in a school of nursing. In 1889 she became head of the newly established Johns Hopkins Hospital in Baltimore, Maryland. Robb served in an administrator capacity, an instructor for students, and wrote a textbook. After a life change (she married), she moved to Cleveland and worked at Case Western Reserve University as a professor of gynecology. She continued to implement innovative ideas related to teaching and learning for nurses. She prompted the development of a hospital economics course, which served as a foundation for nursing. She was a founding member of the International Council of Nurses and a member of the founding committee for the American Journal of Nursing.

Lavinia Lloyd Dock (1858–1956)

Lavinia Dock was from a middle-class family, and she received a proper education in art, music, literature, and language. She saw her mother die at a young age and her father grow ill and not be able to support the family according to its prior financial status. In the late 1870s there was a strong belief that women of her life's station were to be wives and mothers. Throwing convention aside, she looked to nursing as a means of financial security after reading an article regarding a new profession for women in 1882. Dock decided to attend nursing school, even though this was not considered a job for proper young women. She graduated from Bellevue Training School for Nurses in 1886. Shortly after her graduation, she worked to begin a visiting nurse service in New York. In 1887 Dock took a position as the first visiting nurse for a pioneer social organization called the United Workers of Norwich in Connecticut. After being asked to assist with the yellow fever outbreak in Florida by a classmate, she moved to Jacksonville, Florida, in 1888. She eagerly assumed responsibility for care of the sick, and later returned home after two months. Upon her return, she was appointed night superintendent at Bellevue. Even in this position, she continued volunteer relief efforts. During this time Dock authored a textbook called *Materia Medica for Nurses* to promote understanding of compounds used for medicines. She also authored a textbook on hygiene and morality, co-authored the first two volumes, and independently authored the remaining two volumes on the history of nursing. Dock also served as foreign editor of the American Journal of Nursing. In 1890 Dock worked with Lillian Wald at Henry Street Settlement in New York. She realized that the settlement permitted her to utilize her abilities to their fullest. During the 1890s Dock was a member of a group of women at the settlement who focused their efforts on improved education, promotion of nursing organizations, and the creation of a professional journal. This group included Isabel Robb, Adelaide Nutting, and Sophia Palmer. They used the American Journal of Nursing to provide education and information on women's health issues such as venereal disease. She was contributing editor between 1900 and 1923. This journal heightened awareness of women's issues to promote health and wellness. In 1896 Dock worked with Ethel Gordon Fenwick and founded the International Council of Nurses, serving as its secretary from 1900–1922. Dock was an advocate for women's rights.

Mary Adelaide Nutting (1858–1948)

Mary Adelaide Nutting was born in Canada, but entered nursing school in 1889 after reading a newspaper article announcing the opening of the new Johns Hopkins Training School in Baltimore, Maryland. Following her graduation in 1891, she remained at Johns Hopkins as head nurse and was later moved into the position of assistant superintendent of nurses. During that time in nursing's growth and evolution, education was financially supported by hospitals, which used student nurses as cheap labor. This type of educational arrangement did not promote learning as a priority. Students could spend in excess of 60 hours a week working, leaving little time for studying and other educational endeavors. Nutting promoted moving nursing education to universities. Using this philosophy, she limited the number of hours students could perform bedside work in the hospital. In 1907 Nutting accepted employment at Teachers College, Columbia University, and was later appointed as chair of the new Department of Nursing Education. She was the first nurse in the country to be appointed to a university professorship. Her most significant contribution to nursing literature was the first two volumes of *The History of Nursing* that she co-authored with Lavinia Dock. Nutting was a strong supporter of university-based nursing education and contributed many written works, which served to bring focus to nursing education.

Annie Warburton Goodrich (1866–1954)

Annie Warburton Goodrich was born to a family of comfortable means. Due to her family's financial status, she was able to engage in foreign travel and have private tutors for her education. Her first introduction to nursing was seeing her sisters, then later her grandparents, receiving care from a compassionate, knowledgeable nurse. The illness of her father saw the family financial situation take a turn downward. In an effort to be self-sufficient, she entered nursing school. She obtained her nursing education at New York Hospital. Goodrich completed her education and entered the profession as a registered nurse in 1892. Following this education, she obtained a position as head nurse at New York Hospital. She held nurse supervisory positions at Post-Graduate Hospital, St. Luke's Hospital, Bellevue Hospital, Allied Hospital, and Visiting Nurse Service of Henry Street Settlement. She taught in the Department of Nursing and Health at Teachers College in Columbia University. She served for nine years (191–1923) as training school inspector for the New York State Department of Education. Goodrich started the United States Student Nurse Research, now known as the Army School of Nursing. In 1923 she became the first dean of the Yale University School of Nursing. In her lifetime, Goodrich received three honorary degrees. In 1921 she received an honorary degree from Mount Holyoke College (Doctor of Science, ScD), in 1923 she received an honorary degree from Yale University (Master of Arts (MA), and in 1936 she received an honorary degree from Russell Sage College (Doctor of Laws, LLD). Goodrich also served in several professional organizations. She served a one-year term as president of the American Society of Superintendents of Training Schools for Nurses (1905–1906). She was president of both the International Council of Nurses (1912–1915) and the American Nurses' Association (1916–1918). She served as the first president of the Association of Collegiate Schools of Nursing. Goodrich's achievements made a significant impact on the nursing profession.

Lillian Wald (1867–1940)

Lillian Wald was born at a time when city sanitation was minimal or did not exist. As a result, infectious diseases were common. They affected all individuals, regardless of their social standing in the community. It was soon recognized that diseases did not just remain in poor areas, but that rather the plight of all citizens was linked, regardless of financial standing. Communities attempted to address these conditions by hiring trained nurses for home care. Many organizations took up the charge to promote a healthier society. This was the society in which Wald lived and worked.

Wald's interest in nursing stemmed from a family crisis—the illness of her sister who was tended by a private-duty nurse. Following her primary training at the New York Hospital Training School for Nurses, she went to work in a juvenile asylum. She left this position disheartened that nurses had so little influence on the institutional care of these children. This led her to working on the lower East Side of New York based on an identified need for immigrant education in home nursing. An 1893 life experience changed everything for Wald when she visited the home of one of her students in an effort to render care. Her walk "through 'evil' smelling streets, past open courtyard 'closets', up slimy steps of the rear tenement, and finally to the sick room" left her painfully aware of the significant need for reform (Buhler-Wilkerson, 1993, p. 1779). Following this incident, Wald and a fellow schoolmate moved to the neighborhood to work as nurses. Her continued work and solicitation of support allowed her to purchase a house on Henry Street. From this area, she worked to address societal needs that evidenced themselves in disease, poverty, and overcrowding. She pushed for reform from a perspective of health reform and an agenda which included industry, education, recreation, and housing. In 1895 Wald moved into a residence that was to become the Henry Street Nurses' Settlement. She started the Henry Street Settlement out of a community need for health care, education, recreation, and family activities for children and families. By 1910 staff nurses of the settlement were working to address all issues associated with public health, including but not limited to: (a) a milk station; (b) a convalescent home; (c) country homes; (d) first-aid stations; (e) a maternity service and mother-baby health conferences; (f) home visits; (g) several social programs, one of which was a kindergarten; (h) skill classes, which included sewing, carpentry, art, music, dance, etc.; (i) boys' and girls' clubs; and (j) a drama club. This demonstrated Wald's move for social and health reform.

Wald's nursing career is marked by two other innovative initiatives. The next one included insurance coverage for home-based nursing care. She was convinced that home nursing was cost effective and would improve the health of individuals and reduce deaths. This could be beneficial to the insurance company. Following a three-month pilot test by Metropolitan Life insurance company, the program proved to verify this expectation. This relationship proved beneficial to the insurance company and the visiting nurses' association, which received financial support as part of this endeavor. This was the first established national system of insurance coverage for home-based care. Another innovative initiative included the creation of a National Public Health Service. This was called the American Red Cross Public Health Nursing Service. Through this service, standardized public health nursing appeared in small townships across the country. This service kept communities engaged in care with nursing support.

Mary Breckinridge (1881–1965)

Mary Breckinridge came from a prominent family with international influence. Her immediate family included a grandfather who was vice president of the United States, and her father, who was a U.S. ambassador to Russia. Her tutored education allowed her to travel with her family, which exposed her to various cultures and lifestyles. Following the abrupt death of her beloved husband, Breckinridge entered St. Luke's School of Nursing. She remarried and taught French and hygiene prior to becoming a mother to a son and daughter. She lost her second child, a daughter, who was born prematurely. A few years later she lost her firstborn, a son, to appendicitis. Following the death of both children, she and her husband divorced. From these tragedies her life in nursing began. She used nursing as a means of comfort and strength during this time of personal chaos. Breckinridge joined the American Committee for Devastated France after World War I. Following an introduction to nurse-midwives in France and Great Britain, she studied midwifery in an effort to bring this care to the mothers and babies in America. During this time, women in U.S. rural areas had no access to health care, and suffered a high maternal mortality rate. This is where Breckinridge decided to focus her efforts. She established the Frontier Nursing Service (FNS) in 1925 to provide health care to the poor residents of the Appalachian Mountains and eastern Kentucky. These nurses traveled on foot and horseback to care for individuals who lived in these remote areas. She focused her efforts on mothers and on children until the age of one year, but care was extended to anyone seeking it. Money or goods were accepted as payment for individual services. Through speaking engagements and personal connections, she was able to raise millions of dollars to fund the FNS. Through her efforts, both maternal and infant mortality rates dramatically decreased. The FNS staff started the American Association of Nurse-Midwives, which laid the groundwork for the American College of Nurse Midwives. Breckinridge was a pioneer for midwifery and rural health care, and she changed the lives of thousands.

Margaret Sanger (1879–1966)

Margaret Sanger was one of 11 surviving children in a Catholic family. Her mother had numerous pregnancies with some ending in miscarriages. Sanger felt this was the reason her mother was in poor health and that this was instrumental in her death. Seeking a reprieve from the life of poverty she grew up in, Sanger attended school and moved on to study nursing during her educational endeavors. She married and moved to New York, where she became involved in politics and union activities. She worked as a nurse on New York's lower East Side, which a predominantly poor immigrant neighborhood. While promoting help for the sick, she saw many women who had undergone abortions by individuals who were ill-educated or poorly equipped to perform these procedures, as well as women who tried to self-terminate their pregnancies. These situations resulted in significant suffering and disfigurement. In an effort to get health information to individuals who desperately needed it, Sanger started a monthly feminist publication called *The Women Rebel,* which was mailed to constituents. At that time it was illegal to forward information of this nature through the mail, as it was considered "obscene and immoral materials," according to the Comstock law. Sanger fled the country rather than face a five-year prison term for this action. She went to England, where she continued her work for women's "birth control" (a term she coined) rights. In England she was able to research other forms of birth control, which she later smuggled back into the United States in 1915 upon her return, following dissolution of charges against her. She continued her work in the United States by touring to promote birth control, and opened the country's first birth control clinic. Sanger was arrested nine days following the opening of the clinic, which resulted in serving 30 days in jail. After appealing her conviction, the law was amended to permit doctors to prescribe contraception to their female patients for medical reasons. In 1921Sanger established the American Birth Control League, precursor to Planned Parenthood. Sanger immersed herself in women's rights and worked to make it legal for doctors to freely distribute birth control by starting the National Committee on Federal Legislation for Birth Control. A big victory occurred in 1936, when import permission was given by the U.S. Court of Appeals for birth control devices and related materials to be brought into the United States. Sanger was instrumental in establishing the International Planned Parenthood Federation in 1952. She was the impetus for research that resulted in the approval of the first oral contraceptive approved by the Food and Drug Administration in 1960. During Sanger's lifetime, birth control was made legal by the Supreme Court for married couples in 1965, which stemmed from the legal case of Griswold v. Connecticut. These were huge milestones for women's rights.

A Move Toward Licensure

Nursing's evolution paralleled that of other professions. Prior to Nightingale's era, no credentials were available for individuals who called themselves nurses. Certificates of completion were the first credentials given to nurses early in nursing's professional development. Nursing programs varied in length, and some were as short as six weeks while others extended to three years. Some programs had little true education classes, consisting mainly of apprenticeship-type work. This was an issue that nurse leaders addressed in 1893 in a meeting at the Columbian Exposition in Chicago. The American Nurses Association (ANA) evolved in 1896 from this work. A formal directive to addressing this issue came from the ANA, when they proposed permissive licensure for nurses. This concept did not require that all nurses be licensed, but did regulate the use of the title "registered nurse." Only nurses who met the standards for permissive license requirements determined by the state could use this title. It did not restrict use of the word nurse. Anyone could still call themselves a nurse.

During the early 1900s, nursing practice individual identification was merely a list of individuals who had been trained to carry out nursing activities. In 1903 North Carolina was the first state to enact permissive license legislation. This was on the heels of the 1900 initial release of the *American Journal of Nursing*, which merged the efforts of nurse leaders Lavinia Dock, Mary Davis, Mary Adelaide Nutting, Sophia Palmer, and Isabel Hampton Robb. This further served to identify credibility to nursing. By 1923, some 20 years later, all remaining states had permissive licensing for registered nurses. This was just a first step. Nurse leaders desired to take this a step further by requiring mandatory licensure. This would further protect citizens by clearly identifying individuals who had successfully completed the strenuous program of study and met state requirements for licensure. The first mandatory licensure legislation was enacted in 1947 in the state of New York. This landmark action legally protected use of the term "registered nurse." The National League for Nursing (NLN)

Table 1. Women in Nursing

Women in Nursing	Lifespan	Contributions
Florence Nightingale "Lady with the Lamp"	1820–1910	She worked to improve the care of soldiers during the Crimean War and laid the foundation for mastering a body of knowledge specific to nursing through her publication, Notes on Nursing: What It Is and What It Is Not.
Hannah Anderson Ropes	1809–1863	From her political activity and connections during the abolitionist movement, she was able to get changes made to improve sanitation and the appalling conditions in field hospitals for soldiers.
Dorothea Lynde Dix 1976 ANA Hall of Fame Inductee	1802–1887	She was a champion for the mentally ill and those in prison. She traveled from state to state working in jails and almshouses, making organized notes, and petitioning the state legislatures throughout the United States to improve conditions. She was able to successfully get laws and funding imposed to ameliorate living conditions. She also implemented the first nursing dress code.
Susie King Taylor	1848–1912	Born a slave, she traveled with her husband's all-black army unit, caring for the wounded and teaching them to read and write. She became president of the Woman's Relief Corps.
Mary Ann Bickerdyke Mother to the Boys in Blue	1817–1901	She enlisted volunteers to provide needed services, such as washing, cooking, and wound care to soldiers. She provided care alongside the medical care in both the field hospitals and at the frontline during a time when women were not allowed in all-male war camps.
Clara Barton Angel of the Battlefield	1821–1912	Her organizational efforts of locating and documenting the disposition of soldiers in battle became known as the American Red Cross.
Linda Anne Judson Richards 1976 ANA Hall of Fame Inductee	1841–1930	She was the first graduate of the New England Hospital for Women and Children nursing program. She was instrumental in setting up a nurse training school at Boston City Hospital. She also set up the first patient record system.
Mary Eliza Mahoney 1976 ANA Hall of Fame Inductee	1845–1926	The first black woman to hold a nursing position in the United States. Her excellent work in providing nursing care paved the way for other black nurses to obtain a nursing education. She became a lifetime member of the National Association of Colored Graduate Nurses (NACGN).
Isabel Adams Hampton Robb 1976 ANA Hall of Fame Inductee	1860–1910	She was a founding member of the International Council of Nurses and a member of the founding committee for the American Journal of Nursing.
Lavinia Lloyd Dock	1858–1956	She wrote one of the first nursing textbooks. She was a noted author and made significant contributions to nursing literature. She served as foreign editor of the American Journal of Nursing.
Mary Adelaide Nutting 1976 ANA Hall of Fame Inductee	1858–1948	She made significant contributions to nursing through her advocacy of university-based nursing education. She was the first nurse to be appointed to a university professorship.

Annie Warburton Goodrich 1976 ANA Hall of Fame Inductee	1866–1954	She developed Yale University's first nursing program, later becoming its dean. This program later became the Yale Graduate School of Nursing.
Lillian Wald ANA Hall of Fame Inductee	1867–1940	She worked and solicited support to provide home nursing care and addressed societal needs. These public health efforts led to establishment of the National Public Health Service. This was later called the American Red Cross Public Health Service.
Mary Breckinridge 1982 ANA Hall of Fame Inductee	1881–1965	She was a pioneer for midwifery and rural health care. She established the Frontier Nursing Service (FNS) in 1925, which laid the groundwork for the American College of Nurse Midwives.
Margaret Sanger 1976 ANA Hall of Fame Inductee	1879–1966	She fought for women's right to birth control in the United States and abroad. She opened the first U.S. birth control clinic. She established the American Birth Control League, the precursor to Planned Parenthood. Instrumental in establishing the International Planned Parenthood Federation in 1952, she was the impetus for research that afforded approval for the first oral contraceptive by the Food and Drug Administration in 1960.

assumed responsibility for administering the initial nationwide State Board Test Pool Examination in 1950 to validate individual proficiency and knowledge of registered nurses. Today, all states and territories require licensure for anyone who practices as a registered nurse.

Summary

Throughout the course of wars—the Civil War, Spanish-American War, and World War I, nurses played a major role in caring for the sick, injured, and dying. They cared for soldiers and the many afflicted by disease, such as the influenza epidemic in 1917. These women have been of white and African American heritage. Many of these women crossed historical paths. Their years of service overlap, which demonstrate the many changes occurring in the evolution of nursing during these years. There were no men reportedly directly involved in the evolution of nursing, but they served to support many of these women through contributions and appointments to various offices. This acknowledgement allowed them to earn recognition, which further served to promote nursing (see Table 1). These nurses were but a few of the many who served to foster nursing and lay the groundwork for the nurses of today. They worked in broad areas of nursing and rendering aid to those in need.

References

Adventure of the American Mind. (2007). Nursing licensure. Retrieved from http://aam.govst.edu/projects/scomer/student_page1.html

American Nurses Association. *Annie Warburton Goodrich (1866–1954)*. Retrieved from http://www.nursingworld.org/AnnieWarburtonGoodrich

American Nurses Association. (2011). Dorothea Lynde Dix (1802–1887) 1976 inductee. Retrieved from http://www.nursingworld.org/LaviniaLloydDock

American Nurses Association. (2011). Lavinia Lloyd Dock (1858–1956) 1976 inductee. Retrieved from http://www.nursingworld.org/LaviniaLloydDock

Brumgardt, J. R. (1980). *The Civil War Nurse: The Diary and Letters of Hannah Ropes*. Knoxville: The University of Tennessee Press.

Buhler-Wilkerson, K. (1993). Bringing care to the people: Lillian Wald's legacy to public health nursing. *American Journal of Public Health*, 83(12): 1778–1786.

Bullough, V. L. (2002). Isabel Adams Hampton Robb. Retrieved from http://www.nurseweek.com/news/features/02-07/robb.asp

Butchart, R. E. (2010). Susie King Taylor. The New Georgia Encyclopedia. Retrieved from http://www.georgiaencyclopedia.org/nge/Article.jsp?id=h-1097

Castelenova, G. Mary Breckinridge (1881–1965). Retrieved from http://www.truthabout-nursing.org/press/pioneers/breckinridge.html

Cedar Hill Foundation (2011). Annie Warburton Goodrich (1874–1954). Retrieved from http://cedarhillfoundation.org/notable-residents/annie-warburton-goodrich/

Daisy, C. A. (1991). Historiography: Searching for Annie Goodrich. *West J Nurs Res*, (13(3): 408–413. doi: 10.1177/019394599101300310

Dorothea Dix. (2005). Retrieved from http://www.civilwarhome.com/dixbio.htm

Frontier Nursing Service. (n.d.) History of Frontier School of Midwifery and Family Nursing. Retrieved from http://www.frontiernursing.org/History/History-FSMFN.shtm

Gandet, L. (1907). Brothers Hospitallers of St. John of God. In *The Catholic Encyclopedia*. New York: Robert Appleton Company. Retrieved New Advent: http://www.newadvent.org/cathen/02802b.htm

Hospitaller Brothers of St. John of God. (n.d.) Origins of the order. Retrieved from http://www.stjohnofgod.org/origins.html

Johnson, B. M., & Webber, P. B. (2009). Theory and Reasoning in Nursing (3rd ed.). Philadelphia: Lippincott Williams & Wilkins.

Linda Richards. (2010). Retrieved from http://www.nurses.info/personalities_linda_richards.htm

Lux et Veritas. (2008). Annie Warburton Goodrich, 1866–1954. Retrieved from http://www.med.yale.edu/library/nursing/historical/deans/goodrich.html

Mary Eliza Mahoney: First African-American Graduate Nurse. (2011). Retrieved from http://www.essortment.com/mary-eliza-mahoney-first-african-american-graduate-nurse-63922.html

Margaret Sanger. (2011). *Biography.com*. Retrieved from http://www.biography.com/people/margaret-sanger-9471186

Maryland Women's Hall of Fame (2001). Mary Adelaide Nutting. Retrieved from http://mdarchives.us/msa/educ/exhibits/womenshall/html/nutting.html

New York State Senate. (n.d.). Linda Richards. Retrieved from http://www.nysenate.gov/story/linda-richards

Ridgway, S. (2011). Mary Adelaide Nutting, Johns Hopkins School of Nursing. *Working Nurse.* Retrieved from http://www.workingnurse.com/articles/ Mary-Adelaide-Nutting-Johns-Hopkins-School-of-Nursing

Their Stamp on History. (2009). Mary Breckinridge (1881–1965). Retrieved from http:// www.stamponhistory.com/articles/article.php?article_id=6

Truglio-Londrigan, M., & Lewenson, S. B. (2011). *Public Health Nursing from Application to Practice.* Sudbury, ME: Jones and Bartlett Publishers.

Chapter 2: Nursing's Move Toward Professionalism

Nursing's professional status has been a point of inquiry, discussion, and debate for many years. Often, nurses hear the term "professional" in conversation, but fail to truly understand the meaning of the word. Individuals also enter nursing and do not understand the attributes that constitute a professional identity. The term most often referred to when speaking of attributes is profession—a derivative of the term professionalism. Although many definitions have been offered for the term profession, many exhibit similarities and agree that it is an occupational group with a designated set of attributes and/or behaviors. Individuals who enter a profession often do so based on what they identify as their calling, or attitudes driven by commitment rather than profit. There is a service perspective adopted by those entering a profession that focuses on helping others. Upon entering a profession, individuals develop characteristic attributes and attitudes, inclusive of ways of thinking (e.g., the nursing process) to special attire (e.g., nurse's uniform) that allows others to recognize them as being a member of their specific profession. Huber (2010) identified three characteristics found in many definitions of a profession, which include service, specialized education, and a practice based on autonomy. Despite research and opinion, there is no clear definition of what constitutes a profession. This controversy extends to nursing, which continues to struggle with whether it meets the standards of a profession.

Occupation: Nursing's Beginning

Occupations usually began as simple, basic survival tasks. From these tasks, individuals progressed to skilled laborers. These skilled laborers learned their trade through repetitive task performance or under the tutelage of a master tradesman. Several professions evolved from these simple beginnings. The first identified professions were law, medicine, and the ministry.

Individuals even today work in occupations where they learn by doing and perform tasks that are assigned based on knowledge learned on the job. They do not consider this their life's work and seek employment to achieve a specific goal (e.g., a student who works in the fast-food industry while going to college). They work under the supervision of another person and accept the philosophical base of the occupation in which they work (e.g., the customer is always right; make the customer happy). Nursing has evolved from its early pre-Nightingale days, where simple tasks were performed to a technologically based entity. There is a distinct difference between an occupation and profession in several categories. See Table 1, which compares an occupation to a career.

Characteristics of a Profession

Abraham Flexner was a professional educator who identified specific characteristics to describe a profession in a 1915 paper about social work. This work became known as the Flexner report. It is a classic piece of literature regarding professional characteristics and was the impetus for medical education reform. This benchmark report is often used to form the educational foundation for professional status in disciplines.

Table 1. Occupation versus Profession

Category	Occupation	Career
Longevity	Temporary; frequently changing jobs.	Lifelong.
Educational Preparation	May have minimal training; on-the-job training	University/professional degree program based on a foundation of core liberal arts.
Decision Making	Guided by experience or trial and error	Based on evidence validated through research.
Continuing Education	Only what is required for a job or achieved for financial incentive.	Lifelong learning with continuous efforts to improve knowledge base, skills, and abilities.
Level of Commitment	Varies. May be short term and job related to attain personal needs.	Long-term commitment to the profession and its organizations.
Motivation	Self-interest. Work viewed as a means to an end.	Service oriented. Work viewed as a service to society.
Accountability	Lies with supervisor or employer.	Lies with the individual.
Level of Engagement	Work is supervised by others.	Works autonomously.
Expectations	Reasonable work for reasonable pay; work activities performed during specified hours.	Activities related to work extend beyond the boundaries of work hours. Will accept additional responsibilities that promote the good of society, which includes volunteering for organizational or community activities.
Values and Beliefs	Often adopts values and beliefs of employing organization.	Develops values and beliefs that transcend organizational boundaries and become part of the individual's personal life.

Flexner's 1915 criteria stipulate that the following must be present in order for a discipline to be considered a profession:

1. Professional activity is based on intellectual action accompanied by personal responsibility.
2. A profession is based on a body of research knowledge that is continuously expanded.
3. There is a practical application and it is not just theoretically based.
4. Techniques are taught through specialized education.
5. There is an internal organizational structure with members who have a group consciousness.
6. Members are motivated by altruism (an unselfish desire to help others), working in some sense for the good of society.

Flexner identified intellectual endeavor as the first criterion. This relates to individuals who use critical and analytical reasoning in a professional capacity. A professional practice is based on a body of knowledge derived from experience and research. This knowledge base is founded on research evidence to validate and alter care activities. Nurses use the nursing process as a basis for critical thinking and decision making. They progress in their knowledge base as they gain experience in their area of practice. Nurses use evidence-based knowledge or research to validate care activities and establish better patient outcomes (see Box 1: Use of Ventilator Bundles to Reduce Ventilator-Acquired Pneumonia). Evidence-based practice is a significant part of the profession of nursing.

In 1971 Ronald M. Pavalko offered eight dimensions to describe a profession. This scale allows professions to exhibit various degrees of these attributes and possess most, if not all, of these dimensions. An occupation would exhibit none of these dimensions. Professions would exhibit high quality in the work that results from engagement and demonstration of these traits. These can be correlated to nursing. Nursing as a profession has some degree of all dimensions, with some certainly being at higher levels than others.

1. <u>Theoretical framework as a basis for practice</u>. Nursing is based on many theories that are borrowed from other disciplines, and some are adapted to fit the professional perspective. As a result, these theories have evidence-based knowledge that could not have been advanced by the profession alone. Through educational growth and preparation specialists, nursing theories have evolved, adding to the profession's theoretical framework for practice.
2. <u>A profession has relevance to social values</u>. From a historical perspective of nursing through today, nursing has exhibited altruism with a focus on service to others. Nursing focuses on treatment of illness and the promotion of health as part of its goal. Nurses concentrate on patient education as part of these health promotion activities and serve as wellness coaches and managers to promote social values.

Title:	Adherence to Ventilator-Associated Pneumonia Bundle and Incidence of Ventilator-Associated Pneumonia in the Surgical Intensive Care Unit
Authors:	Dorothy Bird, MD; Amanda Zambuto, NP; Charles O'Donnell, MS, RRT; Julie Silva, RRT; Cathy Korn, MPH, RN; Robert Burke, MA; Peter Burke, MD; Suresh Agarwal, MD
Objective:	The objective of this quantitative retrospective study was to examine the impact of adherence to a ventilator-associated pneumonia (VAP) bundle on the incidence of VAP in two surgical intensive care units (SICUs).
Setting:	This study was conducted on two SICUs at a tertiary care (specialized consultative care) academic level 1 trauma center.
Intervention:	The Institute for Healthcare Improvement VAP bundle was instituted at study initiation which consisted of (1) head of bed elevation greater than 30 degrees, (2) daily break from sedation, (3) daily extubation readiness assessment, (4) peptic ulcer prophylaxis, and (5) deep vein thrombosis prophylaxis. A daily checklist was used to verify compliance with all five components.
Outcome Measures:	Patients were assessed for VAP and staff members were assessed for compliance with the initiated VAP bundle.
Results:	Prior to initiation of the bundle in the SICUs VAP was identified in 10.2 cases out of 1,000 ventilator days. Compliance with bundle use increased over the three year study period resulting in a reduction of VAP from study beginning to end. Overall compliance increased from 53% and 63% to 91% and 81% in each SICU. The VAP rate decreased to 3.4 cases out of 1,000 ventilator days. VAP is an expense for any organization and this study identified an estimated cost savings of $1.08 million.
Conclusion:	VAP bundle initiation is associated with a significant reduction in the incidence of VAP in patients in the SICUs. This reduction is accompanied by a financial savings. Initiation of a VAP bundle is an effective method to reduce VAP with continued compliance.

Reference: Bird, D. B., Zambuto, A., O'Donnell, C., Silva, J., Korn, C., Burke, R., Burke, P., & Agarwal, S. (2010). Adherence to Ventilator-Associated Pneumonia Bundle and Incidence of Ventilator-Associated Pneumonia in the Surgical Intensive Care Unit. *Arch Surg. 2010;145(5):*465–470.

3. **A profession has a training (educational) period.** Nursing includes both a theoretical and practice component which was promoted by Nightingale. The educational process for the nurse focuses on establishing the knowledge base needed to practice evidence-based patient management. This process serves to progress scholarly endeavors that continue to advance the profession. The educational base for nurse preparation varies, and this has been the point of much debate. The diverse methods for entry into nursing practice will undoubtedly continue for many years to come.

4. <u>Elements of self-motivation address the way in which the profession serves the patient or family and larger social system</u>. Nurses work to service patients, families, and society at large. Through work in health care organizations, they directly serve these entities. Political activism is another way to translate social values into action. By working with government groups to develop social policies, they expand this objective beyond specific health care organizations.

5. <u>Members are autonomous and control their profession</u>. Nurses do not function totally autonomously. Nurses work under both professional and legislative control in performing their work. Nurses' functions are based on the Nurse Practice Act, which identifies professional practice standards for their respective states. They are also governed by their State Board of Nursing.

6. <u>A profession has a commitment to lifelong work</u>. Many individuals who select nursing as a career see this as their life's work. This is not a means to an end or a mechanism for moving into another profession outside of the nursing arena.

7. <u>Members have a common identity and distinctive subculture</u>. Professionalism is a social phenomenon in which members of the professional community assume some manifestation of a common identify and common destiny. The fate of the individual and the fate of the profession are intertwined.

8. <u>A profession has a code of ethics</u>. The first official *Code for Professional Nurses* was adopted in 1950 by the American Nurses Association. As the profession has evolved, it has been revised to address issues that affect nursing.

This translates visually into a continuum model that demonstrates movement between an occupation and a profession for each dimension. This model is represented below in Table 2.

In 2000 a pharmacy Task Force on Professionalism wrote a paper that derived from five years of study and work. Their goal was twofold: (a) to raise awareness; and (b) lead action on professionalism. The task force defined a profession as "an occupation whose members share 10 common characteristics" (Task Force on Professionalism, 2000, p. 97). They specifically identified characteristics of a profession as:

1. Prolonged specialized training in a body of abstract knowledge.
2. A service orientation.
3. An ideology based on the original faith processed by members.
4. An ethic that is binding on the practitioners.
5. A body of knowledge unique to the members.
6. A set of skills that forms the technique of the profession.
7. A guild of those entitled to practice the profession.
8. Authority granted by society in the form of licensure or certification.
9. A recognized setting where the profession is practiced.
10. A theory of societal benefits derived from ideology.

From: Task Force on Professionalism, 2000, p. 97.

Table 2. Occupation-Profession Model

Dimensions	Occupation		Profession
1. Theoretical framework as basis for practice	Absent	⟷	Present
2. Relevance to social values	Not relevant	⟷	Relevant
3. Training (education) period A	Short time frame	⟷	Long time frame
B	Not specialized	⟷	Specialized
C	Involves items of no symbolic value	⟷	Involves items of symbolic value
D	Subculture not important	⟷	Subculture important
4. Motivation	Self-interest	⟷	Societal interest
5. Autonomy	Absent	⟷	Present
6. Commitment	Short term	⟷	Long term
7. Sense of community	Low	⟷	High
8. Code of ethics	Low development	⟷	High development

Source: Adapted from Pavalko, R. M. (1971). *Sociology of Occupations and Professions.* Itasca, IL: F. E. Peacock Publishers.

The Task Force continued its efforts and defined a professional as "a member of a profession who displays the following 10 traits" (Task Force on Professionalism, 2000, p. 97). These traits of a professional are:

1. Knowledge and skills of a profession.
2. Commitment to self-improvement of skills and knowledge.
3. Service orientation.
4. Pride in the profession.
5. Covenantal relationship with the client.

6. Creativity and innovation.
7. Consciousness and trustworthiness.
8. Accountability for his/her work.
9. Ethically sound decision making.
10. Leadership.

From: Task Force on Professionalism, 2000, p. 97.

In order to display professionalism, the person must actively demonstrate these specific traits of the professional. These traits are promoted through professional socialization which is instilled during an educational process. Professional socialization is not a static process— it involves active engagement of the individual. The individual then adopts and demonstrates the profession's attitudes, values, and behaviors.

Professionalism Concepts from a Nursing Perspective

Conceptual models and investigations of professionalism by nurse investigators have not been a prolific topic. Individuals who have contributed significant information include Lucie Kelly and Barbara Miller

Barbara Miller developed a model in 1984 that has been used in nursing research studies that investigated professionalism. The Miller Wheel of Professionalism in Nursing was developed from socialists such as Hall and Friedson's previous works and from the ANA's policy statement and the Code of Nurses. This visual model can help nurses determine what behaviors Miller considered important to demonstrate professionalism in nursing. Behaviors include participation in professional organizations; being self-regulatory or autonomous; developing, using, and evaluating research; engaging in continuing education to maintain competence; performing community service; developing, using, and evaluating theory; adhering to a code of ethics for nurses; and having publications and communication. These behaviors are depicted as spokes on a wheel that center around nursing education. See Figure 2.

Lucie Kelly compiled characteristics for nursing professionalism in 1981, which reflected themes from prior works. These foundational dimensions carry forward to nurses practicing from the time of identification into today's electronic age of care delivery. These characteristics consist of the following:

1. Services provided are vital to humanity and society's welfare.
2. There is a special body of knowledge that is continually grown through research.
3. Services offered involve intellectual activities and they are accountable for these activities.
4. Practitioners are educated in institutions of higher education.
5. Practitioners are relatively independent and have control of their policies and activities.

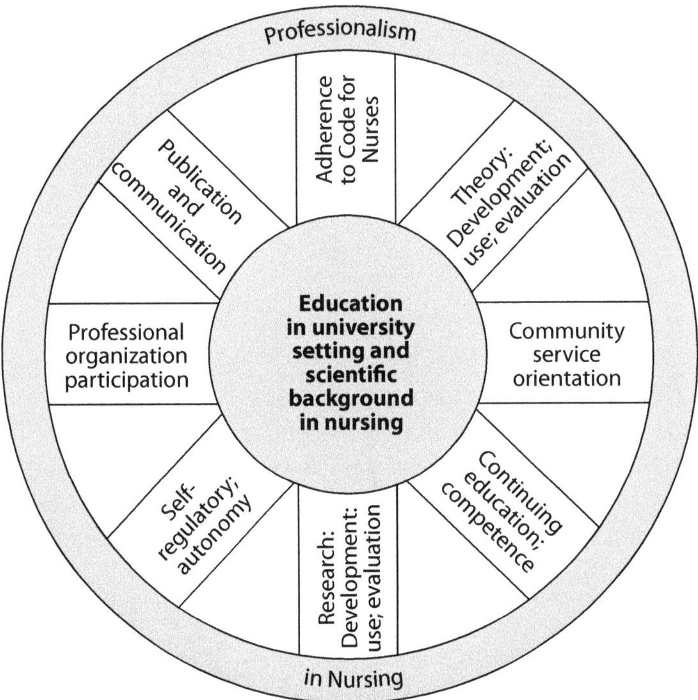

Barbara K. Miller, "A Model for Professionalism in Nursing (figure)," *Today's OR Nurse*, vol. 10, no. 9. Copyright © 1988 by Slack, Inc. Reprinted with permission.

Figure 2. Miller Wheel of Professionalism in Nursing.

6. Practitioners are altruistic (service motivated) and consider this important in their lives.
7. A code of ethics guides practitioner decision making and conduct.
8. There is an organization that encourages and supports high standards.

Components for professionalism that are presented individually by Flexner, Pavalko, the Task Force, Kelly, and Miller are presented in Table 3 in an effort to provide a quick review and comparison.

There are many similarities among the presented professionalism models and concepts. It is difficult to grasp the similarities and differences even viewing these authors side by side. In an effort to add clarity to your understanding, these areas have been delineated based on their conceptual components or themes. Many themes carry through all professional characteristics identified. These include education, service, organization, and ethics. Four of the five authors address altruism and research. Autonomy and theory follow in order of frequency, with three out of five authors identifying this concept as a basis for professionalism. Unique skills and society-granted authority are only identified by the Task Force (see Table 4) which uses the numerical listings from Table 3 for each author.

Challenges to Nursing Professionalism

Professionalism in nursing has not been without its challenges from inception to today. These challenges include educational preparation, diversity in the nursing population, lack of leadership skills, and the nature of the job. It is only through identification and continued work to resolve these conflicts that nursing will proceed to gain the full recognition and respect of a profession.

Educational Preparation

In speaking with many individuals inside and outside of the nursing profession, the first challenge identified is the level of entry into the profession. There is a variety

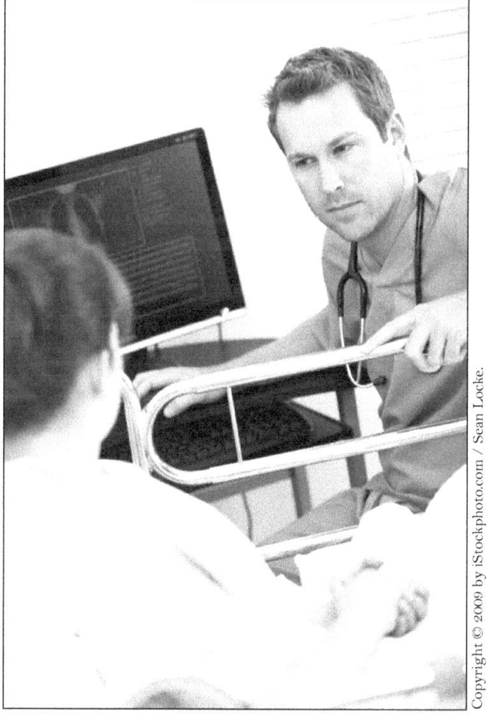

Figure 1. Men serve a vital function in the delivery of competent nursing care to clients, families, and communities.

Table 3. Professionalism Characteristics by Author

Flexner	Pavalko	Pharmacy Task Force on Professionalism	Kelly	Miller
1. Professional activity is based on intellectual action accompanied by personal responsibility.	1. Theoretical framework as a basis for practice.	1. Prolonged specialized training in a body of abstract knowledge.	1. Services provided are vital to humanity and society's welfare.	1. Participation in professional organizations.
2. A profession is based on a body of research knowledge that is continuously expanded.	2. A profession has relevance to social values.	2. A service orientation.	2. There is a special body of knowledge that is continually grown through research.	2. Being self-regulatory or autonomous.
3. There is a practical application and it is not just theoretically based.	3. A profession has a training (educational) period.	3. An ideology based on the original faith processed by members.	3. Services offered involve intellectual activities and they are accountable for these activities.	3. Developing, using, and evaluating research.
4. Techniques are taught through specialized education.	4. Elements of self-motivation address the way in which the profession serves the patient or family and larger social system.	4. An ethic that is binding on the practitioners.	4. Practitioners are educated in institutions of higher education.	4. Engaging in continuing education to maintain competence.
5. There is an internal organizational structure with members who have a group consciousness.	5. Members are autonomous and control their profession.	5. A body of knowledge unique to the members.	5. Practitioners are relatively independent and have control of their policies and activities.	5. Performing community service.
6. Members are motivated by altruism (a desire to help others) working in some sense for the good of society.	6. A profession has a commitment to lifelong work.	6. A set of skills that forms the technique of the profession.	6. Practitioners are altruistic (service motivated) and consider this important in their lives.	6. Developing, using, and evaluating theory.
	7. Members have a common identity and distinctive subculture.	7. A guild of those entitled to practice the profession.	7. A code of ethics guides practitioner decision making and conduct.	7. Adhering to a code of ethics for nurses.
	8. A profession has a code of ethics.	8. Authority granted by society in the form of licensure or certification.	8. There is an organization that encourages and supports high standards.	8. Having publications and communication.
		9. A recognized setting where the profession is practiced.		
		10. A theory of societal benefits derived from ideology.		

Table 4. Comparison of Professionalism Components by Author

Author	Component									
	Education	Service	Organization	Ethics	Altruism	Research	Autonomy	Theory	Unique Skills	Society-Granted Authority
Flexner	#4	#3	#5	#1	#6	#2	——	——	——	——
Pavalko	#3	#6	#7	#8	#2, 4	——	#5	#1	——	——
Task Force	#1	#2, 9	#7	#4	#3	#5	——	#10	#6	#8
Kelly	#4	#1	#8	#3, 7	#6	#2	#5	——	——	——
Miller	#4	#5	#1, 8	#7	——	#3	#2	#6	——	——

of educational backgrounds that mark individual entry into the profession. They are all linked to the term "nurse," from licensed practical nurses to baccalaureate degree nurses. These individuals may be working side by side in a health care organization and identified by a patient to be at the same level on the professional continuum. Educational preparation is one common component of a profession identified by those who have worked to clarity the concept. It stands without argument that professional recognition, status, and power increase with educational preparation.

There is no other profession that allows entry into practice with less than a baccalaureate degree. Many now require master's level preparation in order to be eligible for practice privileges. Nurses are currently prepared at three different entry levels, which include diploma (licensed practical nurse), associate degree (registered nurse), and baccalaureate degree (registered nurse). Discussion of this topic brings about strong reaction from many nurses. This topic has been a divisive issue for the profession over many years and continues to evoke anger and defensive posturing among nurses. Only through a resolution of this issue will nursing evolve into the profession many desire.

Diversity in the Population

Diversity in the nursing population exists on two levels. The first is gender related, and the second is the range of subgroups that exist, which serve to reduce organizational impact. Nursing has historically been equated with the work of women, although there was a time in history where this was not the case. There is a significantly higher number of women in nursing than men. Many male nurses who are in the profession are not at the bedside, reducing the perception of their overall numbers. Many move through bedside nursing to specialties such as nurse anesthesia or nursing administration. Due to the high ratio of women to men in nursing, even with a gradual increase there may never be an equitable distribution of men in the profession. Men serve as a force to change the mode of thinking from women's work to the work of a professional delivering nursing care (see Figure 1).

Men have been part of the nursing profession for decades—as far back as the 11th century in Europe when they were members of religious orders. The number of men in nursing has increased considerably over the last 20 years. The perspective toward men early in the educational development of the school of nursing was to exclude them from entry. Only women were allowed to enroll and thus become nurses. This attitude perpetuated the typical female perspective of the nurse. This perspective gave way to attitudes of men in nursing being effeminate regardless of their sexuality status. This attitude is slowly being overturned as more men enter the profession.

The 2008 National Sample Survey of Registered Nurses reported a total of 2.59 million registered nurses employed in nursing. Of this number, 9.6% were male. Men in nursing were more likely to be older than their female counterparts (median age of 35 for men compared to 31 for women) and work in hospitals. Men made up over 7%

of all employed registered nurses, yet they made up 41.1% of all certified registered nurse anesthetists. The American Assembly for Men in Nursing (AAMN) was established in 1974 to give men a voice in nursing. It has since altered its membership and is now unrestricted and open to all nurses, men and women, in order to address issues in the profession as well as those that are male focused. The AAMN advocates for strengthening and humanizing health care; men to grow professionally and increase awareness of men's contribution to society; continued research, education, and dissemination of information about men's health issues, men in nursing, and nursing knowledge; and support member participation in the nursing profession.

The second diversity issue is that of nursing's division of power through delineation of many subgroups. These groups serve the many specialties in the nursing profession. Many nurses give preference to specialty group organizations like the American Association of Critical Care Nurses (AACN), the Emergency Nurses Organization (ENA), Academy of Neonatal Nursing (ANN), Association of Women's Health, Obstetric and Neonatal Nurses (AWHONN), National Association of Orthopaedic Nurses (NAON), etc. (a listing can be found at http://www.nurse.org/orgs.shtml) and reduce involvement in flagship organizations like the American Nurses Association (ANA) that cross all specialties and represent nurses regardless of their specialty affiliation. Although the ANA is the largest nursing organization in the United States, it has fewer than 10 percent of the 3.1 million nurses reported in 2008. This significantly reduces the power in numbers that could benefit the organization and the nursing profession.

Lack of Leadership Skills

Nursing is a people-intensive profession. Emerging leaders often lack confidence and skill to manage conflict in real-time fashion. They are uncomfortable in discussing and mediating conflicts on all levels—patient and provider. They are not aware of leadership frameworks and theories that promote successful decision making. They are not knowledgeable about interpersonal skills that lead to personal mastery and fail to engage in self-discovery, self-improvement, reflection, and renewal to build a firm foundation upon which to build.

Nursing leaders are needed to empower, motivate, inspire, and influence those around them. Through effective communication and interpersonal skills, they can promote a healthy work environment. A healthy work environment occurs from the support and engagement of the nurse leader. Effective leaders are accessible and play a key role in giving a voice to the issues and concerns of staff to improve patient care environments and subsequently staff and patient satisfaction. They are honest in their dealings with all individuals and expect this in return. They are futuristic in their views and are willing to take risks to see future successes. In order for these successes to be realized, the nursing profession must increase effective education of future leaders in their educational program.

Communication Skills

Communication is essential in nursing—from nurse to patient and from nurse to colleague. Communication is a basic skill and must be cultivated and learned. Many educational programs do not place as much emphasis on this skill as others that are hands-on (e.g., vital signs, assessment, etc.). Communication is not standardized in nursing educational offerings. As a result, there is variability in educational approaches related to content, level, and provision of training for this skill.

Nursing is a communication profession. Nurses must give information on a frequent basis to other health professionals as well as patients and families. Nurses must also deal with individuals from various clinical and life situations. Problems have been identified in nursing communication with older people, those with sexually transmitted diseases, oncological (cancer) patients who may have end-of-life issues, and unconscious patients or those with altered sensorium. These communication problems may result in incomplete information communicated to health care providers during care situations or nursing hand-off following shift completion. These problems may also reduce the amount of patient teaching information due to nurse reluctance and discomfort. These problems in communication may result in human and financial consequences.

Nature of the Job

Nursing has many challenges on a professional level due to the nature of the work involved in patient care. Nurses may work long hours (12-hour shifts), have health care risks, have an increased emotional load due to dealing with individuals in various stages of grief, and death and dying. The length of this work is extensive and List 1 identifies just a small portion of the actual work of the nurse.

List 1. Nature of Nurse Work

- Delivers care in various settings, including physical, mental, and emotional delivery.
- Manipulates patients in the delivery of care activities, including movement (transfer and mobility challenges from full manipulation for patients confined to bed to assistance with patients requiring minimal ambulation assistance).
- Participates in team management and decision-making conferences.
- Collaborates and coordinates planning and implementation of patient care with individuals from other disciplines.
- Develops individualized plans of nursing care.
- Assesses current health status to identify care needs.
- Implements appropriate nursing measures in the delivery of patient care.
- Interprets plans of care developed by others providers for initiation (e.g., physician orders).
- Delegates appropriate care activities to other care providers.

- Supervises others in the delivery of patient care.
- Observes and validates patient outcomes resulting from interventions for patient needs.
- Provides counseling, guidance, and education to patients and families.
- Initiates appropriate referrals and follow-up services for patients and families.
- Records and reports patient health status and other necessary information to health care providers.
- Encourages patient self-care and understanding of current health status.
- Interprets organizational policies, objectives, and services for patients and families.
- Assists in development of organizational policies and procedures.
- Assumes leadership roles.

Nursing shift work varies, based on organizational structure. Some are structured in 8- or 12-hour increments, with 12 hours being a prevalent practice. Hours can range from early morning to late evening (7 am–7 pm), while others are structured in traditional 8-hour shifts (7 am–3 pm, 3 pm–11 pm, and 11 pm–7 am). Shift work can have an impact on sleep, well-being, performance, and outcomes (patient and organizational). Studies have identified that shift work can affect circadian sleep cycles, family interactions, and social life. There is also evidence that shift work increases the risk for significant behavioral and health-related morbidity associated with sleep disorders that can occur.

The nature of work in nursing is fluid, and changes based on setting (area of acute care setting), geographic location (rural or urban), state of practice (related to the Nurse Practice Act), and societal norms and expectations. The nature of nursing work is in a constant state of change due to these and other changes in the health care system, organizational structures, and emerging practice challenges.

Summary

Attitudes and behaviors that characterize a profession cannot be learned through reading and study alone. These must be actively acquired through the process of professional socialization that starts at the beginning of the professional education process. Nursing recognized this early in its educational developmental process, and many programs offer professionalism courses at or near the beginning of their academic program of study. These concepts are then carried out through didactic and clinical courses. Following the academic time frame, these will then be transferred into clinical practice. These include "being good and doing good" as a health professional. Bruhn (2001) identifies 12 pointers for professionals to review and adhere to in an effort to promote professionalism in health professionals (see Table 5). By being committed to these and adhering to standards of the profession, nurses can establish value and reward, which will be reflected in daily patient care activities.

Table 5. Twelve Pointers for Professionalism

Pointer	Expanded information
Be civil.	Treat people with respect. You do not have to like or agree with an individual to treat them as you would want to be treated.
Be ethical.	Stand up for personal and professional standards. Do what is right and not what is expected.
Be honest.	Be forthright and do not participate in gossip or rumor.
Be the best.	Strive to be better than good.
Be consistent.	Behavior should coincide with values and beliefs.
Be a communicator.	Invite ideas, opinions, and feedback from patients and colleagues.
Be accountable.	Do what you say you will do and follow up on issues.
Be collaborative.	Work in partnership with health professionals in related disciplines for the patient's benefit.
Be forgiving.	Everyone makes mistakes, so give people a fair chance.
Be current.	Keep knowledge and skills up to date.
Be involved in the profession	Be active at local, state, and national levels.
Be a model.	Your own words and actions reflect your profession.

From Bruhn, J. G. (2001). Being good and doing good: The culture of Professionalism in the Health Professions. *Health Care Manager*, 19(4); 47–58.

Despite much work that has been done to validate nursing as a profession, much of society continues to view it below this. In order to promote internal and external perceptions of nursing as a profession, nurses themselves must come to terms of agreement on how to define their profession. Nurses continue to take on tasks that are directed to other individuals in the health care organization when there is a need, regardless of its level of duty. They are called on to fill voids that remain when other jobs are unfilled (e.g., the job of housekeeping on shifts when these individuals are reduced in staffing and patient beds must be cleaned for pending admissions). The profession has a ways to go in order to achieve the level of respect attributed to other professions (e.g., physicians, lawyers, and clergy). This will only be achieved through self-promotion to individuals who are at the helm of health care in the United States. This includes health insurance organizations, policy makers, and the public at large.

References

Adams, D., & Miller, B. K. (2001). Professionalism in nursing behaviors of nurse practitioners. *Journal of Professional Nursing.* 17(4): 203–210.

American Association of Critical-Care Nurses. (2005). *AACN standards for establishing and sustaining healthy work environments: A journey to excellence.* Retrieved from www.aacn.org/WD/HWE/Content/hwehome.pcms?menu=Practice&lastmenu

Bird, D. B., Zambuto, A., O'Donnell, C., Silva, J., Korn, C., Burke, R., Burke, P., & Agarwal, S. (2010). Adherence to Ventilator-Associated Pneumonia Bundle and Incidence of

Ventilator-Associated Pneumonia in the Surgical Intensive Care Unit. *Arch. Surg. 2010;145(5):*465–470.

Bruhn, J. G. (2001). Being good and doing good: The culture of Professionalism in the Health Professions. *Health Care Manager,* 19(4); 47–58.

Cardillo, D. (2010) *Your First Year as a Nurse: Making the Transition from Total Novice to Successful Professional.* New York: Three River Press.

Chant, S., Jenkinson, T., Randle, J., & Russell, G. (2002). Communication skills: Some problems in nursing education and practice. *Journal of Clinical Nursing,* 11(1), 12–21.

Drake, C. L., Roehers, T., Richardson, G., Walsh, J. K., & Roth, T. (2004). Shift work sleep disorders: Prevalence and consequences beyond that of symptomatic day workers. *Sleep,* 27(8), 1453–1462.

Dworkin, R. (2002). Nursing's Identity Crisis (Society), *The Wilson Quarterly,* September 22, 2002.

Flexner, A. (1915). Is social work a profession? *School Soc,* 1(26):901.

Huber, D. (2010) Leadership and nursing care management. 4th ed. W. B. Saunders.

Kelly, L. (1981). Dimensions of Professional Nursing, 10th ed. New York: McGraw Hill.

Labyak, S. (2002). Sleep and circadian schedule disorders. *Nursing Clinics of North America,* 37, 599–610.

Miller, B. K. (1988). A model for professionalism in nursing. *Today's OR Nurse,* 10(9), 18–23.

Miller, B. K., Adams, D., & Beck, L. (1993). A behavioral inventory for professionalism in nursing. *Journal of Professional Nursing.* 9(5): 290–295.

Miller, B. K., Adams, D., & Beck, L. (1996). Professionalism behaviors of hospital nurse executives and middle managers in 10 western states. *Western Journal of Nursing Research.* 18(1): 77–88.

Pavalko, R. M. (1971) *Sociology of Occupations and Professions.* Itasca, IL: F. E. Peacock Publishers.

Reynolds, W. J., Scott, P., & Jessiman, W. C. (1999). Empathy has not been measured in client terms or effectively taught: A review of the literature. *Journal of Advanced Nursing* 30((5), 1177–1185.

Shirey, M. R. (2006). Authentic leaders creating healthy work environments for nursing practice. *American Journal of Critical Care,* 15(3), 256–276.

Task Force on Professionalism (2000). White paper on pharmacy student professionalism. *J Am Pharm Assoc* 40(1); 96–100.

U.S. Department of Health and Human Services, Health Resources and Services Administration. (2010). The registered nurse population: Findings from the 2008 national sample survey of registered nurses.

Chapter 3: The Health Care Delivery Setting

N urses deliver health care in a variety of settings. These range from organizational delivery within the confines of a designated area, such as acute care hospitals, rehabilitation hospitals, community health centers and clinics, to home care. For optimum care delivery, organizations offer a variety of services or include access to these services. Nurses interact with individuals and other health

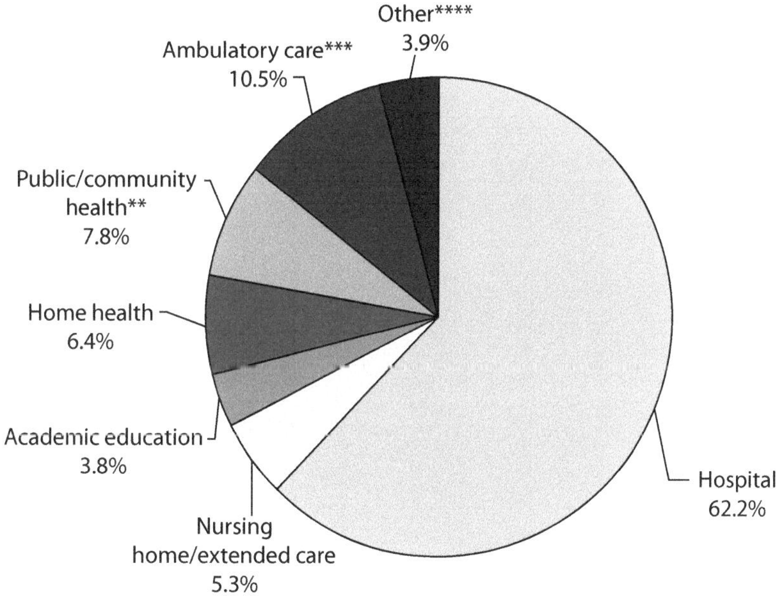

From the U.S. Department of Health and Human Services Health Resources and Services Administration (2010). *The registered nurse population: Findings from the 2008 national survey of registered nurses.* Retrieved from http://bhpr. hrsa.gov/healthworkforce/rnsurveys/rnsurveyfinal.pdf

*Percents may not add to 100 due to the effect of rounding. Only RNs who provided setting information are included in the calculations used for this figure.

**Public/community health includes school and occupational health.

***Ambulatory care includes medical/physician practices, health centers and clinics, and other types of nonhospital clinical settings.

****Other includes insurance, benefits, and utilization review.

Ambulatory care settings employ the next highest number (10.5%) of nurses. Trends for employment settings have changed for nurses (see Figure 2). Between 2004 and 2008, there was an increase in the number of nurses working in hospitals (17.7%) and home health services (68%). There was no significant change in other areas of nursing employment settings.

Figure 1. Employment Settings of Registered Nurses.*

care providers in these settings to promote continuity of care delivery. Patients can move through the system with nurse assistance and guidance. This interdisciplinary approach to the delivery of care works to promote the best outcome for patient and family.

The Nursing Workforce

In 2008 there was an estimated 3,063,162 RNs in the United States, with 2,596,599, or 84%, working in nursing positions. Hospitals employed the greatest number of the RN workforce (62.2%) (see Figure 1).

Types of Health Care Delivery Settings

Acute Care—Hospital Settings

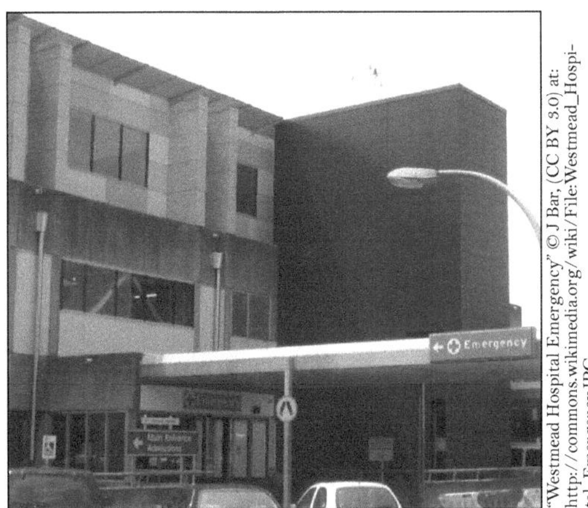

"Westmead Hospital Emergency" © J Bar, (CC BY 3.0) at: http://commons.wikimedia.org/wiki/File:Westmead_Hospital_Emergency.JPG.

    Hospitals offer care for acute situations that require overview and intermittent interventions that would be difficult to obtain in another setting. Hospitals are generally classified based on their size and specialty. Hospitals can vary in size from 25 beds to more than 2000 beds. Specialty types include general medical/surgical, orthopedic, rehabilitation, chronic disease, various addictions, obstetric/maternity, etc. Facilities are also based on financial status—for profit or not-for-profit. For-profit facilities are investor owned and provide care based on achieving a mean profit for areas of care offered. These organizations usually attempt to focus on those areas of care that are profitable for their geographic area. Not-for-profit facilities are usually those based on principles or voluntary groups like religious or community groups. This does not mean that they do not have a positive profit margin. The not-for-profit status

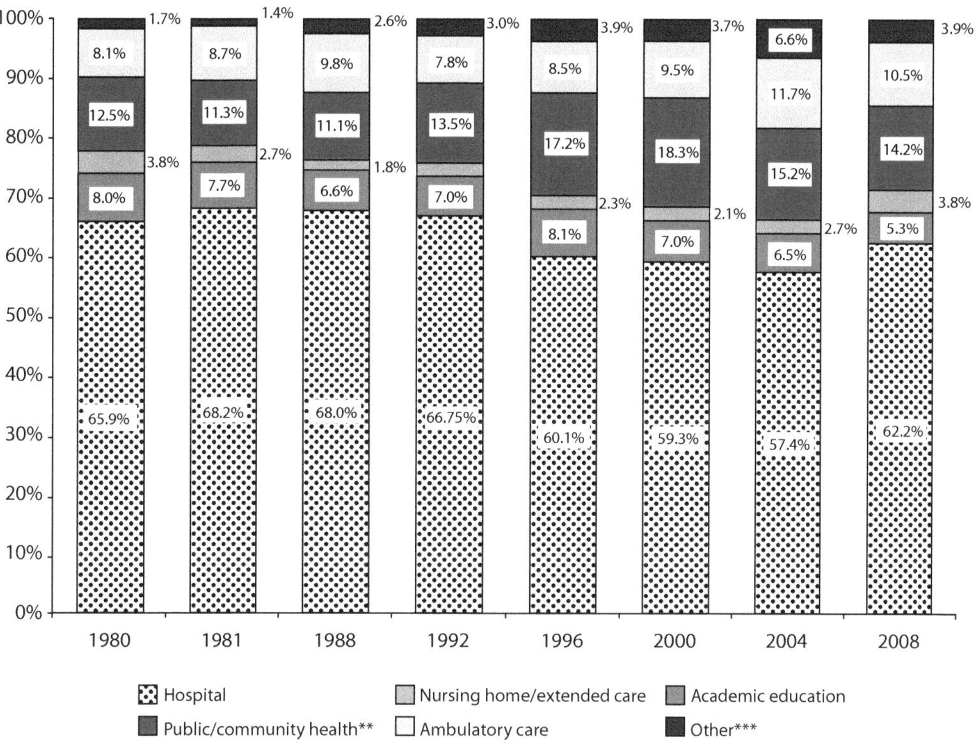

*The total percent by setting may not equal the estimated total of all registered nurses due to incomplete information provided by respondents and the effect of rounding.
**Public/community health includes school health, occupational health, and home health.
***Other includes insurance, benefits, and utilization review.
From the U.S. Department of Health and Human Services Health Resources and Services Administration (2010). The registered nurse population: Findings from the 2008 national survey of registered nurses. Retrieved from http://bhpr.hrsa.gov/healthworkforce/rnsurveys/rnsurveyfinal.pdf

Figure 2. Employment Settings of Registered Nurses, 1980–2009.*

sets limitations on the distribution of profits, the ability or inability to receive donations that are tax deductible, and tax exemptions. All facilities that are not heavily subsidized by government funds or private donations must have a profit in order to remain viable in health care.

Many acute care facilities are accredited in an effort to be eligible for federal grants and o work with educational programs. This accreditation is offered by the Joint Commission, which has a vision of safe, high-quality, best-value care. Additional information may be retrieved from http://www.jointcommission.org/. Joint Commission accreditation is considered to be an indication of status and verification of quality. Nurses working in these organizations during accreditation site visits work within the organizational goals and objectives to achieve a successful outcome.

Some organizations have also achieved Magnet Recognition. This program recognizes health care organizations that have achieved a high level of quality care, excellence in nursing, and nursing practice innovations. Consumers identify

Magnet designation as validation of high-quality nursing care. Magnet Recognition was developed by the American Nurses Credentialing Center (ANCC). Goals and guiding principles for the Magnet Recognition Program® are to "promote quality in a setting that support professional practice, identify excellence in the delivery of nursing services to patients/residents and disseminate best practices in nursing services" (from http://www.nursecredentialing.org/Magnet/ProgramOverview. aspx). Characteristics of Magnet organizations include low RN turnover (<11%), nurse longevity (average of nine-plus years of employment), a high number of RN decision makers with graduate degrees (44%–59%), many nurses certified by a nationally recognized organization (27%–33%), and a high number of nurses with bachelor/university degrees (40%–56%) (from http://www.nursecredentialing.org/ CharacteristicsMagnetOrganizations.aspx). Many nurses desire to work in these nurse-focused organizations.

At least 60% of nurses work in acute care facilities which are open 24 hours a day, seven days a week. They offer orientation or internship periods that may range from a few weeks for general care areas to several months for specialty care areas. Working in this type of facility, whether for profit or nonprofit, allows the nurse to identify an area that appeals to their personal interest and move within the same organization, which can be beneficial for continuity of benefits and longevity. Benefits for the nurse to remaining within the same health care organization include eligibility for educational benefits and the ability to transition up a clinical ladder (a multistep program that begins with entry staff positions and progresses in identified steps based on experience, education, and certification). Salary and position eligibility increase as one progresses up the ladder. Nursing responsibility also increases with subsequent steps.

Private Practice Settings

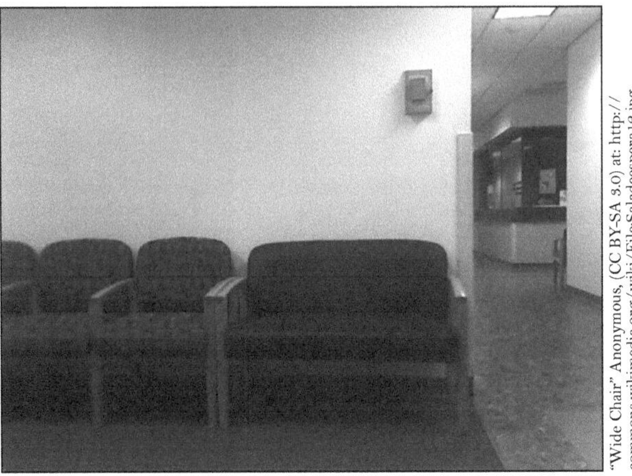

Private practice settings where patients are serviced for acute or chronic conditions may be owned by physicians or nurses. Nurses in private practice are nurse practitioners or clinical specialists. They may be the only health care provider in a designated area. They usually work under protocols and may be in contact (either telephone or electronic) with a physician for additional health care information. These nurses may diagnose illnesses, admit patients to health care facilities, refer patients for further diagnostic treatment or immediate care intervention to a hospital, and/or prescribe medications as needed by patients. Nurses in these situations function within their scope of practice based on their state of residency and/or practice. These nurses own or manage their practice as a business venture and must continue to balance care and financial obligations. Nurses who own their own businesses must manage: employees and all situations that accompany this responsibility (payroll, contracts, tax deductions, etc.); appropriate business taxes; advertising their services; fees for services offered; and patient records maintained in a confidential manner. This responsibility list may be increased by activities that involve collaboration with state or federal organizations or academic institutions. Nurse-owned private practice settings are usually owned by nurses with graduate degrees. They may have nurses as employees to assist with office management and patient care activities. Nurse employees who work in these settings may work variable hours. These offices may offer eight or ten daytime work hours with no or minimal weekend work hours. These offices are often closed on major holidays.

Ambulatory Care

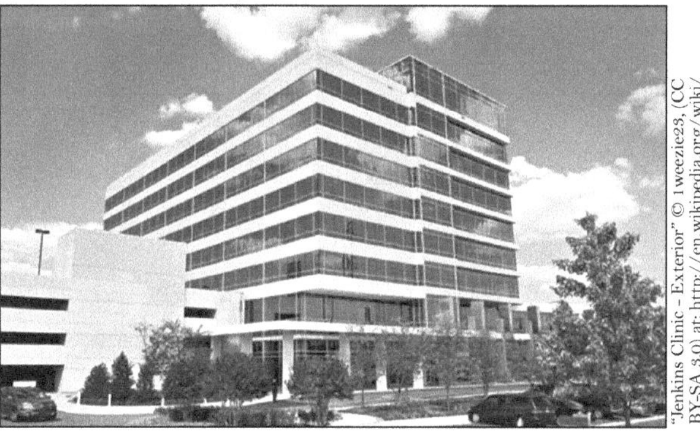

Ambulatory care organizations offer services that, prior to 1980, were mainly in acute care facilities. Some of these centers include surgicenters, emergicenters, wound care centers, pain clinics, childbirth centers, and anticoagulant centers. These allow consumers to select a specific center based on need and pay for this one specific service.

With changes in technology and procedures for surgical intervention, many only require the attention of a nursing care provider for a short duration. Surgicenters offer surgical interventions that do not require overnight hospitalization. Nursing care focuses on postoperative care, including recovery from general anesthesia or other type of anesthetic intervention, based on the type of surgical intervention. Following recovery from anesthesia, wounds are redressed if necessary or ordered and family members are allowed at the bedside. Areas for recovery usually have several stretcher-type beds (beds that are not permanent but rather allow transport from one area to another) separated by curtains for patient privacy. An important part of this type of nursing care is patient and family education regarding care of the surgical area and additional recovery components (pain management, diet, and activity). Patients must meet certain criteria for discharge and are often taken to a waiting vehicle by wheelchair. Usually within 24 hours after the procedure, an additional responsibility of a nurse is patient follow-up.

Emergicenters may be part of a hospital or housed in a separate building in an independent area of the city or town. These centers usually treat acute nonurgent problems. If individuals present to an emergicenter and are in need of urgent care at a hospital, they may be transferred to a hospital facility. These centers may be housed in facilities with designated hours (shopping centers or malls) or be in buildings that allow individual hours of operation. Nurses working in these areas may work various hours and have flexible schedules, with work hours from 1 to 10 hours. These centers require nurses with triage skills and the ability to quickly problem solve in managing urgent situations.

Centers and clinics that offer specific services include wound care centers, pain clinics, childbirth centers, and anticoagulant centers. Wound centers treat chronic non-healing wounds that require additional intervention by a professional individual. These types of wounds can include decubitus (pressure) ulcers or wounds in individuals that have altered circulation (foot wounds in diabetic patients). Pain clinics specialize in managing care and medication for patients who experience chronic pain. The source of their pain can be from any number of situations such as back pain or athletic injuries, and can affect any part of the body. Childbirth centers offer an alternative to home or hospital deliveries. These provide family-centered care in a non–hospital setting. All of these centers and clinics offer varying experiences for the nurse. They allow the graduate nurse an opportunity to work in an area of interest. Some require experience, but others are willing to orient and mentor the new graduate in an effort to facilitate their transition into the specialty area.

Hospice care is focused on end-of-life care. This means that it promotes improving the quality of a patient's last weeks or months of life. Hospice care reflects a holistic philosophy, meaning that it works to address issues related to the whole person. The American Nurses Association (ANA) copublished "Hospice and Palliative Nursing: Scope and Standards of Practice with the Hospice and Palliative Nurses Association." They identify that hospice care provides evidence-based physical, emotional, psychological, and spiritual care to individuals and their families during times of imminent life-limiting illness. According to the Scope and Standards document, hospice is designed to promote quality of life by addressing the relief of suffering throughout the end-of-life course. Hospice nurses work with patients and their families from identification of the imminent end of life, through death, and the family bereavement period.

Hospice care is divided into four basic types based on their central location: hospital; home health agency; skilled nursing facility; or independent. The first three types are usually located within larger organizations. The last, or independent, type is entity- or corporate-owned and separate from any other health care organization. Many hospices offer a mixture of care, including home care and care within a facility. Hospice care can also be given in a home setting outside of any organized facility. Hospice care involves collaborative care between health care professionals (physicians, nurses, social workers, pharmacists, occupational therapists, nutritionists, speech therapists, bereavement coordinators, and pastoral services), family members, and volunteers. Members work within a circle of collaborative care to provide services. Health care individuals may enter and leave the circle based on patient needs.

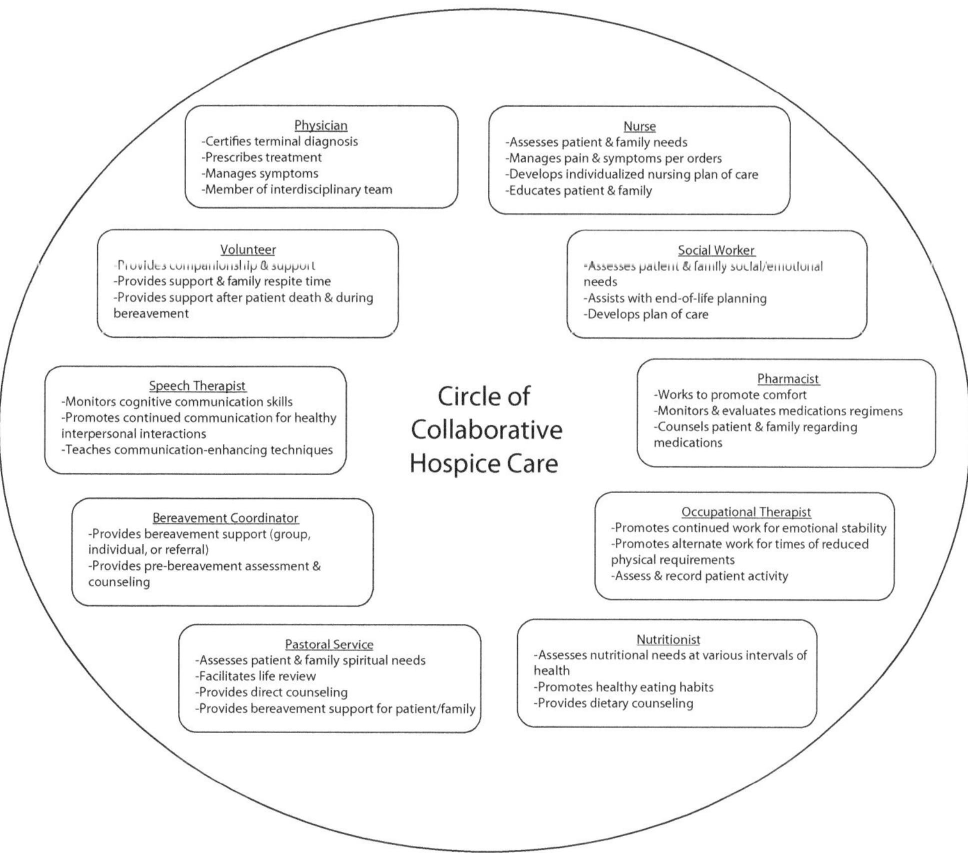

Figure 3. Circle of Collaborative Hospice Care.

Some work techniques by specified health care members and volunteers can be seen in Figure 3. This list is not all-inclusive, because the number and type of individuals involved in the hospice plan of care will differ based on patient need. The goal of hospice care is to give the dying individual comfort, peace, and dignity in the last days, weeks, or months they have remaining to live. It involves a philosophy that includes the patient and family. Family members are assisted in coping with the death and loss of the individual they once knew, as the patient's type of life changes from one of independence to dependence. Family will also ultimately deal with the loss of their loved one. Nurses are an integral part of hospice care. They interact with health care providers, the patient, and family. They often become an integral part of their patients' lives and serve to coordinate care between various types of hospice options (e.g., home care to skilled facility to hospital). Nurses make home or facility visits and serve to notify other members of the collaborative team of situations that may require further intervention. Although hours may not be continuous, working in this type of organization may require varied hours from daytime to evening and night.

Home Health Care

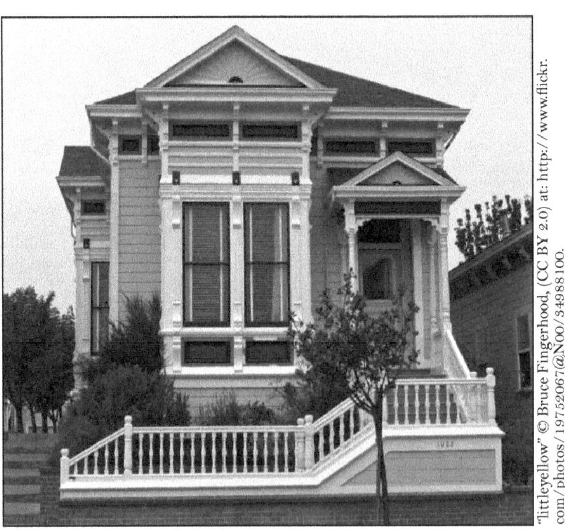

Home health care includes a variety of patient services. Home care services may be given by physicians, home-care aides, nurses, and therapists who collaboratively work to promote out-of-facility care and keep the patient in the home. Home care is a cost effective and convenient type of care. An individual plan of patient care is developed based on needs. This plan will involve addressing (a) needed services; (b) health care professionals to provide the identified services; (c) frequency of needed services; (d) medical equipment needed for effective care or personal activities (e.g., walking [tripod, walker or crutches], toileting needs [high-rise lift on toilet seat or bathroom railing supports], etc.); and (e) expected results from treatment regimens.

Nurses assess patients to identify results from therapies and work to prevent complications such as infections to wounds. They also teach the patient, family members, and friends included in the care circle to effectively implement care activities, recognize complications, and whom to contact for health care problems. Nurses usually work for a specific agency and implement specific physician-approved plans of care. Hours of work may vary from agency to agency and state to state. This type of nursing may require traveling to various counties based on area of coverage by the agency and caseload (number of patients to be seen and type of nursing care to be administered). Confidence in patient management abilities and astute assessment skills are important components of this type of care. Validation of care is essential to reimbursement, so nurses may keep electronic or paper information. Nurses have access to physicians and other health care providers when referral care or specific orders are needed based on patient assessment. As society ages, home health care opportunities are increasing. This type of care is being used to deliver quality, cost-effective health care.

Long-Term Care

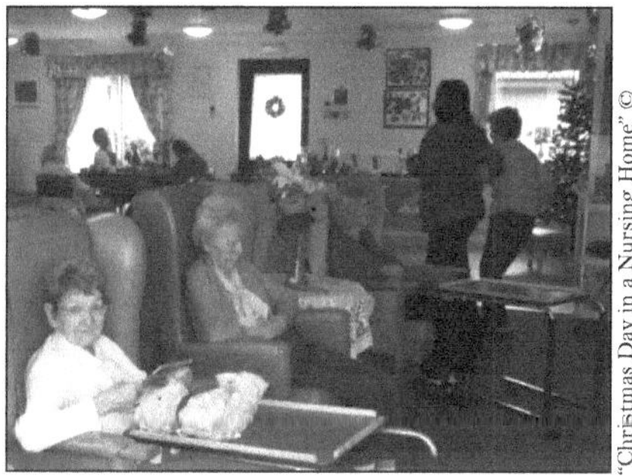

It is estimated that by 2020, 12 million older Americans will need long-term care. This has resulted from innovations in health care that may promote longevity and reduced incapacitation in early stages of recovery. Long-term care is comprised of a variety of services that provide care to individuals with chronic diseases or who have conditions that do not allow for self-care. Long-term care can meet health or personal needs, as these needs can ultimately affect patient health status. Functions provided through long-term care include assistance with activities of daily living, such as bathing, dressing, or toileting.

Long-term care can include institutional care to home care at a variety of levels. Assisted living is one method of long-term care. It offers various levels of care, and is more a social rather than a medical program of care. It offers individuals the opportunity to grow old in their place of residence. Individuals in these facilities often retain control of their care and are given opportunities to retain as much independence as they desire. Assisted living communities are designed to offer variety in care based on personal need. Residents may be assisted with activities of daily living, given reminders regarding medication administration, or given support activity services through enrichment classes such as jewelry making or dance classes. Assisted living can be offered in facilities that are stand-alone buildings or as floors in a continuing-care retirement community building. The physical environment is designed to influence psychological health through a more homelike appearance. The buildings may also be set up in an apartment style with various rooms and layout alternatives, from private rooms to suites. Many assisted living facilities have common areas that are designed for relaxation and comfort, which promote meaningful activities and resident interactions. They may have garden areas and atriums with fireplaces. Some offer central dining areas with pleasant surroundings and entertainment. These state-regulated facilities use nurses based on the degree of care provided. Hours of work can vary and some with in-resident care are set up with shift work like acute care facilities. They may offer eight- to 12-hour shifts. Nurses assess and manage situations related to the residents' health care situation (e.g., wound care for diabetic foot wounds).

The nursing home is a form of long-term care institution. These facilities are not just for older individuals who can no longer manage their own care due to illness or debilitation. These places may offer an alternative to individuals with injuries, acute illnesses, or those needing additional postoperative care with the need to recover outside a hospital. Many nursing homes are set up organizationally like acute care hospitals with limited diagnostic and therapeutic departments. They can offer both long-term and short-term care based on resident need. They may also be affiliated with an acute care facility or hospital with transfer capabilities when a higher level of care is required for residents. The level of skill and expertise offered by nursing homes can vary widely. Some provide a continuum of care for individuals from home care to skilled nursing care. They may have the ability to implement sustainable interventions, such as intravenous (IV) fluids for dehydration, enteral feedings (administration of nutrition through a feeding tube placed through the nose or mouth into the stomach), to maintaining proper nutritional status or oxygen administration to increase circulating oxygen levels in the blood to accelerate activity tolerance. Some nursing homes have subacute or specialty units. A subacute unit offers a continuum of care that may be initiated in an acute care hospital, but at a lower level of intensity while providing needed support, such as rehabilitation. This intermittent care may be provided until the person can return to a prior living arrangement. Specialty units may exist for individuals with: (a) Alzheimer's disease or other forms of dementia; (b) respiratory care needs beyond oxygen administration or for patients who have tracheostomies or are on ventilators (breathing machines) to assist with breathing; or (c) kidney failure needing renal dialysis (the use of a machine to perform the normal functions of the kidneys, such as removal of waste and fluid). Some of these units have residents that require sophisticated, labor-intensive, 24-hour care. Nurses working in subacute units perform care much like that administered in an acute care hospital, but for individuals who need to be maintained instead of having interventional, episodic care. Nurses who work in long-term care facilities enjoy working with geriatric individuals, as many of the residents of these facilities are older. They like the interaction and assistance they can provide individuals as they age. They can work with individuals and their families in managing health situations, administering care, and offering referrals for health care of older individuals.

Summary

Health care delivery offers a variety of settings for nurses to enjoy throughout their professional careers. Many nurses work in various settings until they identify the setting of their choice and preference. This allows them to experience areas that correlate to their preference, related to their work environment (acute to long-term care) and their life situation (full-time work with a family or part-time work while attending a program of higher education).

References

American Nurses Association (2007). Hospice and palliative care nursing: Scope and standards of practice. Silver Spring, MD. American Nurses Association.

Cress, C. J.(2011) *Handbook of Geriatric Care Management.* 3rd ed. Sudbury, MA: Jones & Bartlett Learning.

Joel, L. (1998). Assisted living: Another frontier. *Am J Nurs* 98:7.

Medicare.gov (2009). The official U.S. Government Site for Medicare. Retrieved from http://www.medicare.gov/longtermcare/static/home.asp

The National Association for Home Care and Hospice (2011). *Home care and hospice facts and stats.* Washington, DC: The Associations. http://www.nahc.org/facts/ Retrieved August 28, 2011.

Sharp, N. (1992). Community nursing centers coming of age. *Nurs Manage* 23:18–20.

Sloan, F. A., & Vraciu, R. A. (1983) Investor-Owned and Not-for-Profit Hospitals: Addressing Some Issues. *Health Affairs,* 2(1):25–37. doi: 10.1377/hlthaff.2.1.25

U.S. Department of Health and Human Services Health Resources and Services Administration (2010). *The registered nurse population: Findings from the 2008 national survey of registered nurses.*

Chapter 4: Acute and Chronic Care

Nurses function in care settings that can descriptively be divided into two components based on illness: acute and chronic care. Acute care is care given for an illness that starts abruptly and is usually short-lived. Chronic care is care for an illness that develops gradually and persists for an extended period of time. These concepts will be presented in this chapter in an effort to help delineate care required for the management of individuals in both settings.

Acute Care

Most nurses in health care work in acute care settings. Acute care settings provide outpatient and inpatient care. Individuals who present for care in these settings have conditions or situations that cannot be addressed in an office or clinic. Some individuals require care that cannot be provided in these settings that offer limited medical care. Acute care facilities offer services at higher levels than offices or clinic settings.

What Is Acute Care?

Acute care is urgent health care attention given to individuals experiencing situations that require short-term treatment or intervention. This care is often administered in an acute care facility, which services individuals with a point of entry such as an emergency room or emergency department. Health care interventions for situations that bring an individual to these doors may be brief or extended, based on severity.

Acute care facilities are usually hospitals that have various settings, with services that extend from immediate treatment and discharge to treatment and admission for further care. Acute care institutions offer services that go beyond home treatment and office care. Many acute care facilities offer these services in an effort to allow recovery from an illness or accident. The philosophy of most acute care facilities is treatment to promote recovery and discharge as soon as possible in an effort to reduce costs of care and promote return to society.

Acute care services include but are not limited to the following:

- Medical units (e.g., medical surgical, pediatric, maternity, labor and delivery, etc.)
- Surgical services (e.g., cardiovascular surgery, orthopedic surgery, plastic surgery, etc.)
- Laboratories (e.g., blood chemistry and microbiology, pathology, management of blood products for distribution to other areas of the acute care facility, etc.)
- Radiology (e.g., X-rays of various body parts, ultrasound, computed tomography [CT], magnetic resonance imaging [MRI], etc.)
- Cardiac services (e.g., electrocardiogram, echocardiogram, stress testing, etc.)
- Emergency department
- Pharmaceutical services
- Respiratory services
- Dietary services

Acute care services are generally delivered by individuals specially trained in a specific area. Many services are available 24 hours a day. For services with limited access during night and weekend hours, many can be initiated instantly in the event of an emergency situation that requires intervention services. These services may have reduced numbers of staff in the facility during these hours but have access to other personnel who are capable of responding to an immediate call for specific services. Personnel features include licensed nursing personnel, physicians, dietitians, social workers, rehabilitation specialists, recreation therapists, and pharmacists, to name a few.

Acute care organizations employ the majority of nurses in health care. This is based on the 2008 National Sample Survey http://www.hanys.org/workforce/reports/2010-06-07_nurse_survey_results_2010.pdf

Acute care organizations offer a variety of opportunities for nurses. Although many positions are bedside nursing–based, there are other positions, including supervision of nurses and other health care professionals, education of nurses and the public, or research to improve patient outcomes. Nursing is the largest health care profession according to the *2008 National Sample Survey of Registered Nurses* conducted by the Health Resources and Services Administration (HRSA). At that time, there were more than 3 million registered nurses nationwide with 2.6 million (84%) of all licensed RNs employed in nursing. Of this number, more than half (60%) worked in acute care organizations.

Acute Care Opportunities

Registered nurses working in acute care facilities include nurses educated at the associate degree, baccalaureate degree, master's degree, and/or doctoral degree level. Many new graduates enter the workforce through the acute care- or hospital-based route. Many organizations offer new graduate internship opportunities. These extend orientation timelines to allow the graduate nurse an opportunity to develop skill proficiency and improve critical thinking. This timeline gives the new nurse a safe environment in which to develop coping skills in adjusting to a new profession. These provide the nurse with resources to successfully transition from school to the work environment.

Nurses can also extend their educational bases to promote specialization in the management of individuals requiring acute intervention in hospitals. Nurses working in areas such as surgical intensive care units, coronary care units, burn units, postoperative open-heart surgical units, etc., require specialized knowledge to care for patients in these settings. These patients have a higher acuity level and require an intensive level of care. Critical care units house individuals with serious conditions that require intense nursing management. Nurses working in these specialized areas can increase their knowledge bases through continuing education and higher academic levels of education. Many generalist or specialist certification opportunities exist for nurses working in acute- or hospital-based care organizations. These opportunities extend to medical surgical nursing, critical care nursing, emergency room nursing, neonatal nursing, etc. Acute care organizations offer numerous opportunities for nurses in various areas of patient care in general or specialty positions.

These organizations may offer programs for progressing upward in mobility from entry levels for nurses. These programs provide professional enrichment and growth for nurses. As nurses gain experience, they are able to move beyond the entry level. These often require more components in addition to experience. These components may include continuing education, demonstration of clinical competence in a specific area, obtaining certification in a designated area, or pursuing formal education to achieve a specific degree level (e.g., baccalaureate degree in nursing or master's degree in nursing). As these levels are achieved, nurses are able to move up the rungs or steps of the ladder (see Figure 1).

Responsibility, specialization, and salary increase as the nurses progress up the clinical ladder. There are dual benefits to the clinical ladder concept. These include increased nursing status while continuing to work at the bedside and retention of nurses proficient in care and use of evidence-based research. See Box 1 for an example of how evidence-based research can be used in acute care management.

This leads to better patient outcomes and reduced health care costs. Work hours may also vary based on ladder position of the registered nurse. While many acute care organizations typically maintain 12-hour shifts with variable holiday and weekend schedules, some higher-level nursing positions reduce these hours to be more consistent with eight-hour days, five days a week. Variable shifts may also be available for the nurse at higher ladder positions (e.g., four ten-hour shifts per week, variable eight-, ten-, or 12-hour shifts, etc.). Nurses at all levels in acute care organizations work with patients and families to promote the best outcomes possible and improve the quality of care for patients upon discharge (see Figure 2).

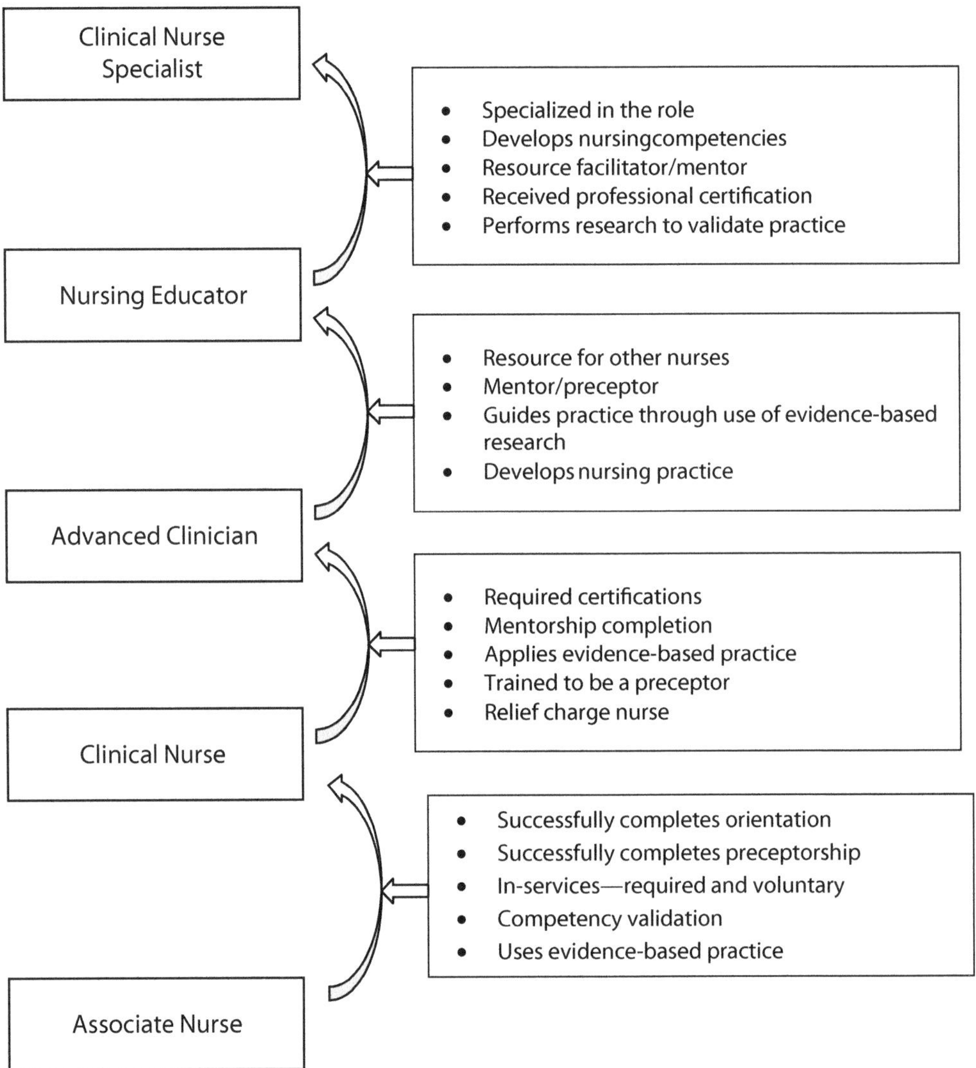

Figure 1. Example of Clinical Ladder with Required Competencies/Activities

Box 1. Use of Evidence-Based Research in Acute Care Management

Title:	Chlorhexidine, Toothbrushing, and Preventing Ventilator-Associated Pneumonia in Critically Ill Adults
Authors:	Cindy L. Munro, RN, PhD, ANP, Mary Jo Grap, RN, PhD, ACNP, Deborah J. Jones, RN, PhD, Donna K. McClish, PhD, and Curtis N. Sessler, MD
Journal:	*American Journal of Critical Care*, 2009, 18(5), 428-438. doi:10.4037/ajcc2009792

Background: Ventilator associated pneumonia (VAP) is an infectious process in the lungs that is directly correlated with the patient being on this breathing device. A risk factor for development of VAP is pathogen transmission from oral flora. During the first 48 hours of intensive care unit admission oral flora undergoes a change to predominantly gram-negative which is more virulent (Abele et al., 1997). Research related to use of chlorhexidine is conflicting and as a result this solution is not a standard of care or used in combination with other bundled components promoted to reduce VAP.

Aim: This study "hypothesized that oral interventions would reduce the incidence of VAP" (Munro et al., 2009, p. 429).

Methods: This was a randomized controlled clinical study where staff members administered one of two interventions based on participant groups. A 2 X 2 factorial design was used to allow for hypothesis testing. With this technique the effect of each intervention and any interaction between intervention techniques could be investigated.

Participants: Participants were recruited from three intensive care units at a medical center. Patients were screened to identify their eligibility to be part of the study prior to recruiting efforts. The sample consisted of 547 individuals who were mostly Non-White males approximately 48 years of age.

Ethical Considerations: The study was fully approved by appropriate ethical committees. Participants were given study information and their consent or the consent of their legally authorized representative was obtained to be part of the study.

Procedures: Study participants were randomized to one of two groups: toothbrushing or use of chlorhexidine.

Data Analyses: Data analysis techniques included descriptive statistics which allowed investigators to identify characteristics of the sample. In order to identify effects for interventions logistic regression analysis was used which compared proportions of patients in each group.

Results: "The toothbrushing protocol did not have a significant effect on VAP" (Munro et al., 2009, p. 435). Chlorhexidine has bactericidal activity that toothbrushing does not possess. Although both toothbrushing and chlorhexidine reduce the number of organisms remaining in the mouth, toothbrushing causes an intermittent reduction insufficient to reduce pneumonia risk. A combination of both toothbrushing and the use of chlorhexidine did not provide a benefit over using chlorhexidine alone.

Conclusion: The study failed to verify that toothbrushing reduced the risk for VAP. Patients in one subset of the study benefited from chlorhexidine use on day three. These patients demonstrated a reduction in their number of oral organisms. Interventions are more likely to have the greatest effect on early VAP if initiated very early in the care regimen related to their ICU stay. This has implications for nursing care.

References used for synopsis:
Abele, H. M., Dauber, A., Bauernfeind, A., et al. Decrease in nosocomial pneumonia in ventilated patients by selective oropharyngeal decontamination (SOD). *Intensive Care Med.* 1997;23:187–195.
Munro, C., Grap, M., Jones, D., McClish, D., & Sessler, C. (2009). Chlorhexidine, toothbrushing, and preventing ventilator-associated pneumonia in critically ill adults. *American Journal of Critical Care*, 18(5), 428–438. doi:10.4037/ajcc2009792

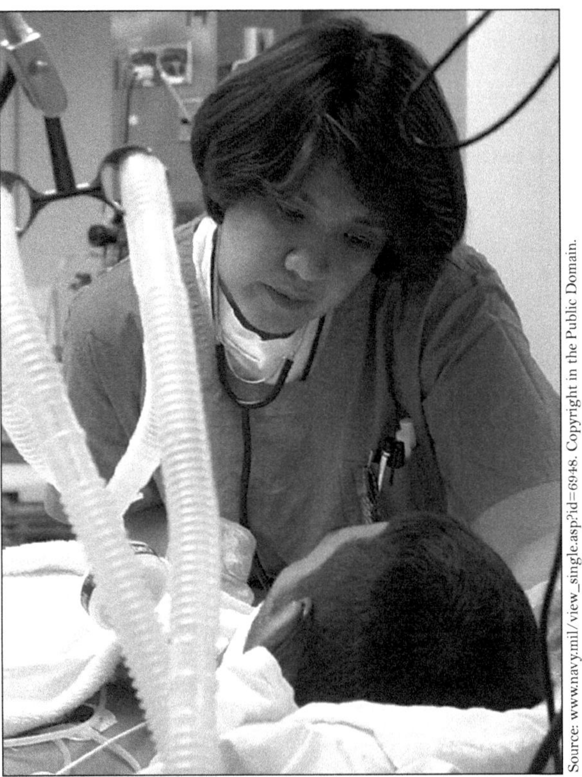

Figure 2. Acute Care/Hospital-Based Nursing Care

Chronic Care

Unlike acute care, chronic care involves multiple interactions with the health care system. This type of care occurs when an individual has a condition that requires intermittent evaluation and/or adjustments to care activities or pharmaceutical interventions. More than 146 million people, or almost one half of the U.S. population, live with some form of chronic illness. There is projected to be more than a one percent increase in this number by the year 2030. This will put the estimated number of individuals with chronic illnesses at 171 million. Patients with chronic conditions may be managed in home setting or extended care based on disease and level of disability.

Nurses play a crucial part in management of the chronic care patient population. Nurses need to have the skills to work within a collaborative system to manage these individuals, as many will have multiple illnesses. These illnesses will include, but not be limited to, diabetes, heart disease, high blood pressure, chronic obstructive pulmonary disease, depression, asthma, renal failure, and many others. It will take skill and interactions in health systems that involve health organizations, community centers, and individual care providers to assist in maintaining the health of these individuals to a state of wellness that will allow them to contribute to their family social system and society. Nurses will need to use evidence-based care initiatives to promote the highest quality of care. Evidence-based care will allow delivery of care that is validated through the research process. See Box 2 for an example of how evidence-based research can be used in chronic care management.

Nurses managing patients in chronic care settings will need to be skilled in patient education. They will need communication techniques that encourage patients to adhere to health care initiatives. It is important for nurses to work with patients to establish goals and objectives that are attainable and focused. Patients will need to learn care activities that promote self-management.

Nurses will need to facilitate coordination of care activities in individuals with chronic diseases. This patient-centered approach will promote individualized care. Individualized care activities will be necessary, since patients will present with various combinations of chronic diseases. This will allow specialized care to utilize interventions that promote the best patient outcomes.

Individuals with chronic diseases may be managed in the home setting, or based on disease severity, be required to stay in a facility with varying degrees of assistance. Chronic care facilities are often referred to as long-term care facilities since these patients are housed in these facilities for extended lengths of time. Chronic care or long-term care facilities offer several levels of care. These levels include: Custodial care for active individuals who require minimal assistance; long-term personal assistance for persons who need more than custodial but less than intensive care; or skilled care, which is the level of assistance required for individuals who need intensive 24-hour care. Persons with debilitating conditions may require assistance but not intensive care and may use facilities called nursing homes, board and care homes, sheltered care homes, or other names which imply care on an extended basis without intensive interventions.

Nurses will need to promote the use of evidence-based interventions to promote quality care outcomes for individuals with chronic diseases. Evidence-based care will support improvements for care at all levels of the chronic fare organization.

The nurse is important in promoting health literacy for patients with chronic diseases. Since many individuals with chronic illnesses present with combinations of diseases, their care can be complex. They are likely to have multiple prescriptions and require interactions with care providers on a more frequent basis. In addition to promoting compliance with visits to health care providers, it is important to promote literacy in facilitating medication adherence (see Figure 3).

Box 2. Evidence-Based Nursing Care in Diabetes

Title:	Lived Experience of diabetes among older, rural people
Authors:	Sharon R. George, PhD, RN, CNL and Sandra P. Thomas, PhD, RN, FAAN
Journal:	*Journal of Advanced Nursing*, 2010, 66(5), 1092–1100.
	doi:10.1111/j.1365–2648.2010.05278.x

<u>Background</u>: Diabetes is taking a devastating toll on lives and quality of life. According to the International Diabetes Federation (2007) it is the fourth leading cause of death worldwide. The U.S. is one of the top three nations with individuals who have diabetes (World Health Organization, 2008). In this country over 23 million people have diabetes with this number significantly increasing by 2030 (American Diabetes Association 2009a, 2009b).

Rural people with diabetes tend to be diagnosed later in their lives (Dabney & Gosschalk, 2009). People with diabetes carry out most of their own care. These people must make daily decisions regarding care activities and education in diabetes self-management is considered critical to improving their choices, promotion of health and reduction of complications and achieving optimum blood glucose levels.

Education of people with diabetes is usually done using lecture content, tests to assess knowledge level and return demonstration of skills. This is used to promote change in individuals regardless of their age. This has been identified as promoting a challenge to the older person who has established years of patterns and behaviors. There are also health status changes that make education of older persons different from that of younger persons. These can include visual problems and cognitive impairment. According to Jack et al. (1999) diabetes education has failed to address the impact [on] individual social circumstances and environmental factors. One significant factor includes the financial status of older persons and the impact this can have on purchasing prescribed medication.

<u>Aim</u>: The aim of this research study was to reveal experiences and perceptions of diabetes self-care as narrated by older people who were insulin dependent and living in a rural area.

<u>Methods</u>: This research study used a phenomenological approach to data collection. This approach allowed for experiences to be captured through verbal interaction for later analyses.

<u>Participants</u>: People who were English-speaking and between 65 to 85 years old and able to willingly speak to researchers were used. In addition, these individuals had to have a diagnosis of diabetes. Individuals who participated in the study included eight African Americans and two White females who lived in rural areas. These women had diabetes between 7 to 39 years and all had visible signs of complications from diabetes.

<u>Ethical Considerations</u>: The study was fully approved by appropriate ethical committees. Participants were given study information and their consent was obtained to be part of the study.

<u>Data Analyses</u>: All interviews were audiotaped and later transcribed verbatim for continued analysis. Transcription accuracy was verified by reviewing conversations while listening to the tapes. Themes related to the lived experiences of the female participants were identified by researchers from the transcriptions.

<u>Results</u>: There were four themes identified from the conversations. These included

1. *'Your body will let you know: If you miss it you'll wind up in a coma'*. This theme identified participant fear related to altered body functions related to their disease. They felt that healthcare providers were not willing to listen to their concerns about these functions and placed them on a regimen of care they could not follow. Participants used words like 'Didn't believe me', 'wouldn't listen', and 'Tried to tell them'.
2. *'I thought I was fine but I wasn't'*. Participants believed they were adequately managing their diabetes, however after the disease progressed they developed irreversible, disabling complications from their diabetes.
3. *'Only way out is to die'*. Participants knew that diabetes was a lifelong disease and they felt that it had taken over their lives. It dictated each day of their lives. They did not perceive any significant improvement in their condition despite traditional healthcare intervention. They accepted the end result of this disease.
4. *'You just go on'*. Despite complications endured by individuals they felt that they were managing their diabetes to the best of their ability. They accepted the limitations of their disease.

<u>Conclusion</u>: Nurses have been educating patients about diabetes from a medical model perspective. This education needs to be approached from a nursing perspective which incorporates the individual's insights and experiences. It is important to incorporate adaptations and modifications based on the individual's perspective and not focused from an intellectual, financial and psychological system. This approach serves to frustrate people and may not improve glycemic control. Focusing on an individual approach would direct interventions to working with individuals who have diabetes to address complications that were troublesome to them and caused the most distress in their self-management regime. This includes planning timely nursing care and emphasizes individualized evaluation of the environment and experiences. This care should be negotiated and collaboratively initiated with the individual.

References used for synopsis:
American Diabetes Association (2009a). Retrieved from http://www.diabetes.org/diabetes-statistics.jsp on 10 April 2009.
American Diabetes Association (2009b). Retrieved from http://www.professional.diabetes.org/CPR on 12 September 2009.
Dabney S., & Gosschalk A. (2009). Diabetes in Rural America: A Literature Review. Retrieved from http://www.srph.tamhsc.edu/centers/rhy2010/Vol2diabetes.htm on 13 April 2009.
International Diabetes Federation (2007). *Diabetes Atlas*. 3rd edn, Retrieved from http://www.idf.org/home/index.cmf?unode on 2 April 2009.
Jack L., Liburd L., Vinicor F., Brody G. & McBride-Murry, V. M. (1999) Influence of the environmental context on diabetes self-management: A rationale for developing new research paradigm in diabetes education. *The Diabetes Educator* 25(5), 775–790.
World Health Organization (2008) Country and Regional Data. Retrieved from http://www.who.int/facts/world_figures/en on 2 April 2009.

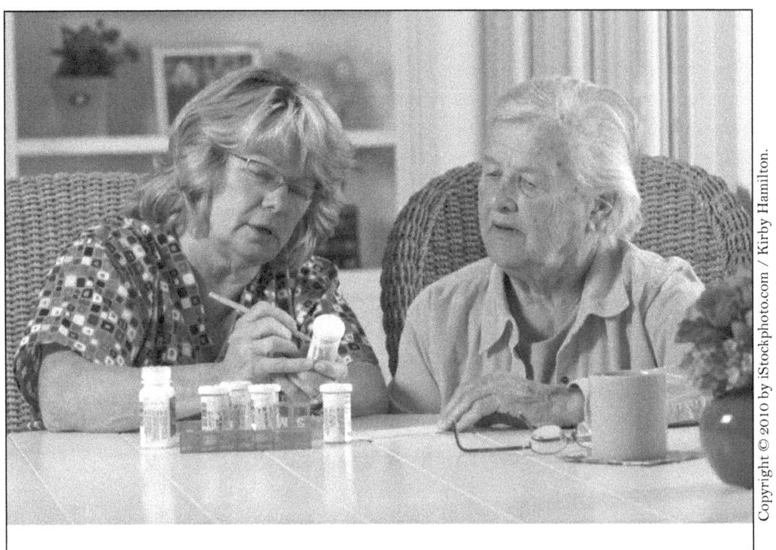

Figure 3. Health Care Literacy in Chronic Care

Health care literacy is the ability of patients to interpret health information in order to make informed choices for care and manage current health situations. Individuals with chronic conditions can have frequent health care encounters that relate to current and new diseases. If patients do not understand their care activities and diseases, they cannot make informed decisions regarding activities that may affect their health. As a result, conditions deteriorate and individuals lose the ability to contribute to society and family goals.

Chronic care management by promoting understanding of care activities, inclusive of medications, is an important component of patient safety. Information should be tailored to the educational level of the individual's health care vocabulary. Explanations that use plain language or enlisting the assistance of an interpreter allow accurate understanding. This fundamental information is important to promote accurate self-monitoring and disease management. Making sure patients have a level of health literacy that allows them to make healthy and informed choices about health care is important. Only through the promotion of patient education and confirmation of a patient's health care literacy level will nurses work to improve quality of life for individuals with chronic health conditions.

Summary

Nursing management of acute and chronic diseases varies. These must be individualized and nursing-focused, directed toward immediate intervention or promotion of self-care. Patients continue to move between these areas of care, and as society ages, this will continue to be a challenge for the nurse as care provider.

References

Abele, H. M., Dauber, A., Bauernfeind, A., Russwurm, W., Seyfarth-Metzger, I., Gleich, P., & Ruckdeschel, G. (1997). Decrease in nosocomial pneumonia in ventilated patients by selective oropharyngeal decontamination (SOD). *Intensive Care Med*, 23:187–195. DOI: 10.1007/s001340050314.

American Association of Colleges of Nursing (2011). Creating a more qualified nursing workforce. From http://www.aacn.nche.edu/media/pdf/NursingWorkforce.pdf

American Diabetes Association (2009a). Retrieved from http://www.diabetes.org/diabetes-statistics.jsp on 10 April 2009.

American Diabetes Association (2009b). Retrieved from http://www.professional.diabetes.org/CPR on 12 September 2009.

Dabney, S., & Gosschalk, A. (2009). Diabetes in Rural America: A Literature Review. Retrieved from http://www.srph.tamhsc.edu/centers/rhy2010/Vol2diabetes.htm on 13 April 2009.

George, S. R., & Thomas, S. P. (2010). Lived Experience of diabetes among older, rural people. *Journal of Advanced Nursing*, 66(5), 1092–1100. doi:10.1111/j.1365-2648.2010.05278.x.

International Diabetes Federation (2007). Diabetes Atlas. 3rd ed., Retrieved from http://www.idf.org/home/index.cmf?unode on 2 April 2009.

Jack. L., Liburd. L., Vinicor. F., Brody. G. & McBride-Murry. V. M. (1999) Influence of the environmental context on diabetes self-management: A rationale for developing new research paradigms in diabetes education. *The Diabetes Educator* 25(5), 775–790.

Munro, C., Grap, M., Jones, D., McClish, D., & Sessler, C. (2009). Chlorhexidine, toothbrushing, and preventing ventilator-associated pneumonia in critically ill adults. *American Journal of Critical Care*, 18(5), 428–438. doi:10.4037/ajcc2009792.

Partnership for Solutions: Johns Hopkins University, Baltimore, Maryland, for the Robert Wood Johnson Foundation (September 2004 Update). "Chronic Conditions: Making the Case for Ongoing Care."

World Health Organization (2008) Country and Regional Data. Retrieved from http://www.who.int/facts/world_figures/en on 2 April 2009.

Chapter 5: Patient Rights

As health care has changed, so have patient rights. Patient rights have been the center of attention in the new electronic age. Nurses serve to support and enhance patient rights while administering quality care. Nurses do this through advocacy activities and adherence to privacy and confidentiality. Nursing care is part of this partnership and included in expectations that are to be fulfilled. Nurses must work to address rights from all perspectives of the organization, those initiated by other health care organizations as well as those promoted by nursing as a profession. This chapter will review patient rights and the nurses' role in promoting care and advocating for patient rights.

Patient Rights and Health Care

Patient rights are those things related to health care that an individual is entitled to in the process of having their health care needs fulfilled. These fundamental rights must be addressed and respected by nurses as their patients navigate through the health care system. Awareness and understanding is imperative to promoting compliance. These patient rights are based on guidelines that include the HIPAA Act of 1996 and on organizations like the American Hospital Association.

Fundamentally, patient rights include the right to make choices in their treatment. As long as the patient is considered intellectually sound, it is important to give factual information in order to promote decisions that are right for them. This goes back to the ethical right to informed consent. Patient options may include medicinal treatment, surgical treatment, radiological, or a combination of any or all of these. The patient also has the right to refuse treatment options. The patient may refuse any or all options for a designated illness. This right can be exercised regardless of the opinions of the health care provider. Patients have the right to make decisions about their own end-of-life care options. This can be done prior to being admitted to any type of organization through an advanced directive. The advanced directive is a legal document regarding end-of-life care. It often includes who can make decisions for the individual when they are no longer able to make such decisions due to illness or continued medication (e.g., continuous pain medication). Each state has its own criteria regarding this type of document and how legally binding it is regarding health care.

It is important for patients to not only have an advanced directive, but to speak with family members and make their wishes known. This will allow family discussion and identification of important care activities that the patient may or may not desire in end-of-life decision making.

It is also important for the nurse to have an awareness of parental rights related to health care for a child (individual under 18 years of age). These rights have continued to change and expand as society has evolved through recognition of minors as individuals. These can vary considerably from state to state. One state may allow minors to be treated for a sexually transmitted disease without parental knowledge, while another may not. There may be times when the wishes of the parents are overturned by the court system. This can occur if the child is believed to be in imminent danger and their life depends on receiving a designated treatment (e.g., a child whose parents refuse to allow the administration of blood due to religious convictions after a trauma has resulted in considerable blood loss, and it is felt that survival depends on blood administration). Some states recognize teenagers 15 years or older as "mature minors," and will occasionally adhere to the wishes of the individual. This variability is the result of debates and various ways of thinking over parental responsibilities, the potential immaturity and vulnerability of children, and emancipation rights of children from parental decisions. Generally, parents are considered legal guardians of their children, and therefore they have the right to make health care decisions. In some cases, parental rights have legally been granted to others and this right passes to them. Many states recognize parental rights up to the age of 12 years for a child. It is the teenage years where this thought differs among states. An "emancipated minor" is an individual who has terminated parental rights, which means that parental consent is not necessary for health care decisions, regardless of severity. The "mature minor" is an individual who is usually over 13 years of age and can provide informed consent through demonstration of understanding of the designated procedure (and the procedure is usually not serious in nature). The "mature minor" status may be implemented when minors request contraception or in some states, sexually transmitted disease treatment, as these services are identified as right-to-privacy situations. A state that has a "mature minor" doctrine allows minors to give consent for some medical procedures. This has been seen in more cases with individuals 16 years or older who demonstrate understanding of the designated procedure and the procedure is not serious. The concept has been in use since 2002, and some states have enacted the doctrine as a statute, which means it is law. An example of a state mature minor doctrine is in Box 1.

Nurses also work to promote patient rights identified by the American Hospital Association. This organization has identified six patient care partnership expectations, rights, and responsibilities. These include (a) high-quality hospital care; (b) a clean and safe environment; (c) involvement in one's care; (d) protection of privacy; (e) help when leaving the hospital; and (f) help with billing claims. Specifics related to these rights are identified in Table 1.

Rights are universal and relate to other patient right components such as HIPAA, which has been discussed under the legal aspects of nursing. Fundamentally, patient

Box 1. Mature Minor Doctrine Example

Mature Minor Doctrine, Tennessee

An emancipated minor is someone under the age of 18 who is independent of parental control and support. Legally, an emancipated minor is treated the same as an adult and can make his own health care decisions. He can also appoint a health care agent or surrogate.

For a minor who is not emancipated, the underlying rule is that a physician must get parental (or guardian) consent before rendering medical treatment, except in cases of emergency. However, the legislature and the courts have carved out exceptions to this rule that allow a minor to consent to medical treatment under certain conditions.

By statute in Tennessee, a physician can treat a minor without parental consent for certain health issues, such as drug abuse, venereal disease (STD/STI), contraception, and prenatal care. Also by statute, a physician may render emergency care to a minor without parental consent. After a reasonable effort has been made to contact a minor's parent or guardian, a physician may render emergency medical treatment to a minor without parental consent if the physician has a good faith belief that the emergency treatment is necessary to save the life of the minor or prevent further deterioration of the minor's condition. In Tennessee, an un-emancipated minor cannot obtain an abortion without parental consent or judicial bypass.

The courts in Tennessee have also adopted the "mature minor" doctrine that allows a physician to treat a mature minor without parental consent. In determining who is a "mature minor," Tennessee follows the "Rule of Sevens."

- Under the age of 7 there is no capacity, and the physician must have parental consent to treat (unless a statutory exception applies).
- Between the ages of 7 and 14, there is a rebuttable presumption that there is no capacity, and a physician generally should get parental consent before treating (unless a statutory exception applies).
- Between the ages of 14 and 18, there is a rebuttable presumption of capacity, and the physician may treat without parental consent unless the physician believes that the minor is not sufficiently mature to make his or her own health care decisions.

TN Department of Health
HIV/STD Program From http://health.state.tn.us/STD/PDFs/Mature%20Minor%20Doctrine.pdf

rights are affected by legal and ethical decisions, which can intertwine to make this a complex situation for the nurse.

Advocacy as a Right

The role of patient advocate has been in the functional role of the nurse from the days of Nightingale. The nurse acts as a liaison between the patient and health care providers. The American Nurses Association (ANA) includes the word "advocacy" in its definition of nursing.

Serving as a patient advocate is a means of supporting and promoting patient safety, the right of every patient. The nurse serves to defend the rights of patients when they are at their most vulnerable. They have assisted patients and their families navigate the sometimes complex health care system—not making decisions, but

Table 1. Patient Care Partnership Rights

Right	Explanation
High-quality hospital care	Care delivered with compassion, skill, and respect to the patient when needed, which includes management of pain and the identity of individuals administering care (e.g., students, residents, nursing assistants, physicians, nurses).
Clean and safe environment	Policies and procedures to prevent health care errors, abuse, or neglect. All incidents will be reported to the patient and any resulting changes that may be necessary as a result (e.g., additional tests or procedures required to address problems).
Involvement in one's care	Decisions will be joint between patient and provider and include discussion of medically appropriate choices, treatment plan discussions, identification of health and coverage to promote appropriate decisions, understanding personal health care goals and values, and understanding who should make decision about care when the patient is not able to do so.
Protection of privacy	Confidentiality of the relationship between the patient and caregiver is respected and a notice of privacy is made available that describes the way in private information is used, disclosed, and safeguarded, as well as how a copy of the patient record can be obtained.
Help when leaving the hospital	Community resources will be identified for follow-up care and any relationship between entities (hospital and organization) will be disclosed. Patient education, which includes information and training will be given (e.g., dressing changes needed for wound care, information regarding when to contact a care provider or when emergency care is needed, etc.).
Help with billing	Care organizations will file health insurance forms, including those for private and federal programs (e.g., Medicare and Medicaid). For individuals who do not have insurance, the facility will provide assistance in locating financial help or in making arrangements for payment. Billing questions will be addressed by the organization.

From: Patient Care Partnership Rights, from the American Hospital Association. Retrieved from http://www.aha.org/aha/content/2003/pdf/pcp_english_030730.pdf

promoting understanding in order to assist in an informed decision regarding treatment. Advocacy is not necessarily an innate skill. Nurses may have an introduction to it in their early educational nursing experience, but often learn through identifying and mimicking the behaviors of expert nurses. Advocacy is important to demonstrating that the fundamental nursing concepts of caring underlie the moral value system of the nursing profession. The process of patient advocacy starts with establishing a trusting relationship and works through various steps terminating with upholding patient/family decisions. See Figure 1 for steps in the advocacy process for nurses.

Advocacy in nursing has its theoretical basis in nursing ethics. The ANA's Code of Ethics for Nurses includes the following language in Provision 3, which relates to this function of the nurse. This provision states, "The nurse promotes, advocates for, and strives to protect the health, safety, and rights of the patient." (American Nurses Association, Code of Ethics). The nurse promotes the patient's right to privacy. When administering care, the nurse is responsible for maintaining reasonable privacy of the physical space. This includes visual and auditory privacy. Patients are often exposed during assessments and other care activities or procedures. During assessments and physical examinations, curtains should be drawn, patient room doors closed, and all provisions possible made to maintain no view of the patient by others.

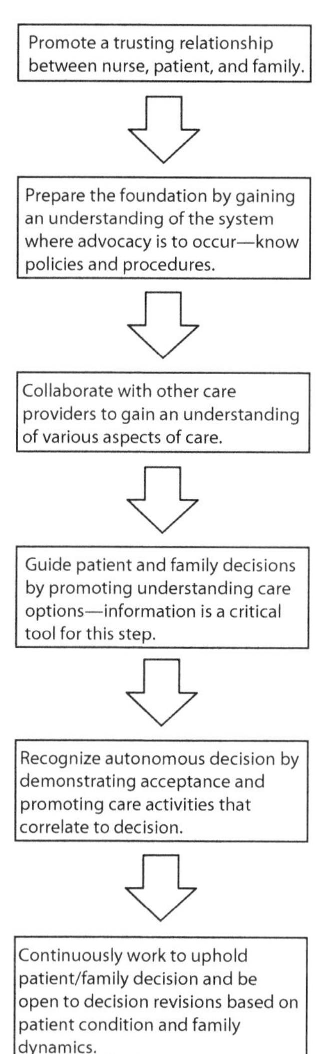

Figure 1. Steps in the Advocacy Process for Nurses

These procedures should be done at a time when visitors are reduced in numbers, or visitors should be requested to step out of the room during these situations. During transport, patients should be covered whether in wheelchairs or on stretchers. Family members should only remain upon request and/or approval of the patient. It is important during exchange of information to ensure that the nurse lowers their voice to prevent accidental information transmission to other care providers, patients, and family members who do not have a need to know. It is imperative that patient information not be accidentally transferred to others. These activities are the responsibility of the nurse.

Some nurses are uncomfortable with the advocacy role as part of their responsibility. The nurse must work through barriers that may occur to promoting this patient right in order to promote patient safety. Barriers may be personal or inter-personal. Personal barriers include discomfort due to inexperience. Working with a mentor who is experienced in promoting advocacy can assist with this personal barrier. Interpersonal barriers can be nurse to patient or nurse to care providers. Establishing a trusting relationship begins with the first nurse-patient encounter. Introductions can present an open perspective of the nurse by encouraging the patient to ask questions and by responding to patient needs as soon as possible. The nurse should listen actively and communicate clear, factual information regarding care to promote understanding by patient and family. Nurse to care provider relationships can be promoted through presentation of self as a knowledgeable, competent professional. Working to complement care of other care providers while performing those tasks identified as nursing responsibilities can assist in promoting a cohesive approach to advocacy for a specific patient and eliminate this interpersonal barrier.

Right to Confidentiality and Privacy

Confidentiality is closely linked to privacy. All patient information is treated in this manner. Only individuals who have a "need to know" are given patient information. Violations of confidentiality and privacy can jeopardize trust and have a negative impact on the nurse-patient relationship. This could result in the patient not disclosing information that could affect safety and progression toward wellness. Transmission of information should be guarded in all methods, verbal, written, or electronic. Some organizations have patient codes for relaying information to family members over the phone. If in doubt, it is better to err on the side of caution when giving phone updates.

It is important to know organizational policy and procedures regarding disclosure of information. Disclosure of information may be required in certain situations. These may specifically relate to situations that address safety. Situations that may require disclosure could include:

- Patient protection from harm or injury—abuse situations
- Safety of others—threats to others
- Public health threat (e.g., anthrax, *Chlamydia trachomatis* infections, diphtheria, gonorrhea, hepatitis, Human Immunodeficiency Virus [HIV] diagnosis, Lyme disease, malaria, measles, mumps, syphilis, tetanus, tuberculosis, etc.)

Health care organizations and entities collect protected and very personal health information. A privacy rule exists that identifies how this information is used by the patient's specific health care provider. These rights must be addressed and individuals must be notified of these rights. These are disclosed in the Notice of Privacy Practices. These rights include the patient's right to: (a) know how personal health information is used in the organization or practice; (b) know who has accessed their information; (c) access their information; (d) request an amendment to or correct their individual health information; and (e) file a complaint about the use of their health information.

Nurses should know policies and procedures related to confidentiality and privacy of information. One place to start is the organization's Notice of Privacy Policy (45 CFR §164.520 through §164.528). Each health care organization is required to describe how information is used for care and statement(s) about individual rights regarding use of the information. The Notice of Privacy must include:

Table 2. Notice of Privacy

Required Inclusions
1. Information about who and for what purpose health information is kept, which includes types of uses for treatment, payment, and health care operations.
2. Descriptions of other uses of information with disclosures that may be made without individual consent or authorization.
3. Other uses of information that is collected, such as appointment reminders, fund-raising purposes, release of information to health care sponsors, and marketing.
4. How patients can access, inspect, amend, or correct their information.
5. Guidelines for filing a complaint about a privacy violation by the specific provider and a notification that the patient can file a complaint with the Department of Health and Human Services.
6. Penalties that may occur for individuals who may violate privacy laws and violations as well as patient confidentiality.

Often patients ask the nurse how to engage components of the privacy notice. Nurses should be familiar with its components. Not adhering to compliance is not only an ethical violation but a legal one as well.

It is important to protect all information regardless of the source or form. Sources of patient information can include obvious and not-so-obvious items. These can include, but are not limited to, the following:

- Copies of paperwork with patient identifying information.
- Laboratory or radiological patient data.
- Pharmacy records of medications dispensed to be administered (medications can give a clue to a patient's diagnosis, such as medication used specifically for the treatment of HIV, Acquired Immune Deficiency Syndrome [AIDS], or a sexually transmitted disease).
- Packages used to dispense medications, such as intravenous medications hung via secondary infusion sets (these medications come with full patient identification for proper identification prior to administration).
- Computer screens used for data entry at the bedside, unit station, or office, or in more public areas on mobile wireless computerized entry components (e.g., Computers on Wheels [COWS], Workstation on Wheels [WOWS]). See Figure 2.

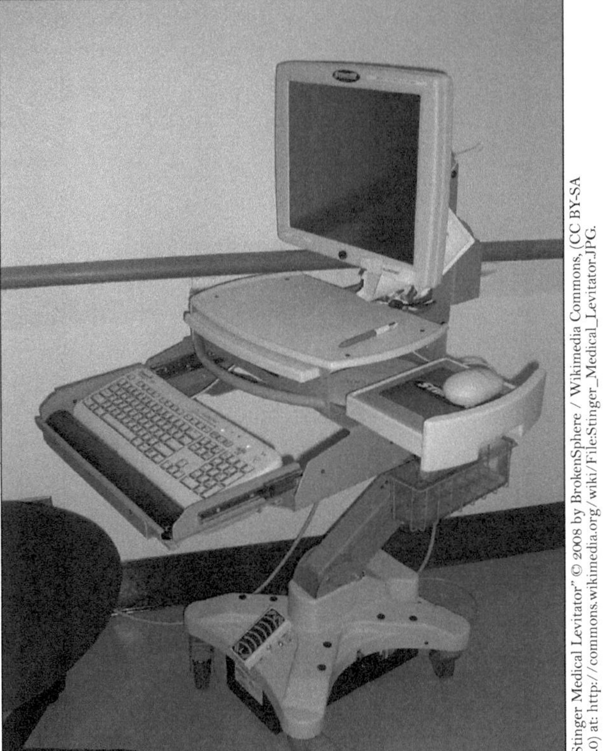

Figure 2. Computer Workstation

- Personal devices for data access or entry (some health care providers have access to patient information via personal computerized handheld devices).
- Surveillance information that may be held in data sets.

Items with patient identifying information should be managed based on the organization's policy. Some require obliteration of identifying information on the object with special markers. There may be disposal in special places for internal or external shredding for security. This can include collection and disposal by special companies who specialize in disposal of sensitive information.

Summary

Nurses are the front line in patient care. As patient advocates and protectors of information, they must be involved in compliance. They must strive to create a work environment where communication complies with laws. The patient care environment must also be structured to reduce the accidental communication of patient information to other individuals who do not have a right to know. Nursing communication habits in the work environment must drastically differ from social interactions. Communication of patient information must occur in a private setting and not a public forum like a busy office setting or an elevator. Nurses should seek private areas for exchange of private patient information such as an empty care room or a place out of earshot of other individuals. This mindset is imperative to maintaining confidentiality of private information and prevention of financial fines and personal sanctions for violations.

References

"Acknowledging the Hypocrisy: Granting Minors the Right to Choose Their Medical Treatment." *New York Law School Journal of Human Rights.* Summer 2000.

American Nurses Association. (2001). *Code of Ethics for Nurses with Interpretive Statements.* Washington, DC: American Nurses Publishing.

Beh, H. G., & Pietsch, J. H. (2004). Legal implications surrounding adolescent health care decision-making in matters of sex, reproduction, and gender. *Child Adolesc Psychiatr Clin N Am* 13. 675–694.

Centers for Disease Control and Prevention (May 13, 2011). Summary of Notifiable Disease—United States, 2009. 58(53); 1–100. Retrieved from http://www.cdc.gov/mmwr/preview/mmwrhtml/mm5853a1.htm

English, A. (2007). Sexual and reproductive health care for adolescents: legal rights and policy challenges. *Adolesc Med* 18. 571–581.

"Informed Consent to the Medical Treatment of Minors: Law and Practice." Schlam, Lawrence.

"Medical Care for Minors: How to Consent to Medical Care for Minors." Available at http://www.cmanet.org/, Aug. 7, 2001.

"Minors and the Right to Consent to Health Care." Boonstra, Heather, & Elizabeth Nash. Available at http://www.agi-usa.org/, 2000.

Office of Disease Prevention and Health Promotion, U.S. Department of Health and Human Services. *Healthy people 2010 leading health indicators.* Available at: http://www.healthypeople.gov/Document/HTML/uih/uih_4.htm

Schlam L., Wood, J. P. (2000). Informed consent to the medical treatment of minors. *Health Matrix: Journal of Law-Medicine,* 10(2):141–174.

Smith, A. P. (2004). Patient advocacy: Roles for nurses and leaders. *Nurs Econ.* 22(2); 8890.

"Standards for Privacy of Individually Identifiable Health Information: Final Rule." 45 CFR Parts 160 and 164. *Federal Register* 67, no. 157 (August 14, 2002). Available at http://aspe.hhs.gov/admnsimp/.

Taylor, P., & Ferszt, G. (1998). The nurse as patient advocate. *Nursing,* 28(8); 70–71.

The Patient Care Partnership. American Hospital Association. Retrieved from http://www.aha.org/aha/content/2003/pdf/pcp_english_030730.pdf

Valvano, T. J. (March, 2009). Legal issues in sexual and reproductive health care for adolescents. *Clinical Pediatric Emergency Medicine*, 10(1), DOI: 10.1016/j.cpem.2009.01.004.

Chapter 6: Problem Solving in Nursing

Problem solving by the nurse is an important foundation to identifying essential patient changes that can affect patient safety in the health care environment. Nurses are the contact liaison between patient and physician or advanced practice nurse. There are key components that facilitate this foundational element for the nurse. It is an integrated component in the educational process—both classroom and clinical components.

Critical Thinking

Critical thinking is considered an essential element in nursing practice and a point of focus in nursing education. There are many definitions of critical thinking (see Table 1).

Table 1. Definitions of Critical Thinking

Author	Definition
American Philosophical Association (APA)	Purposeful, self-regulatory judgment that uses cognitive tools for making judgments. These cognitive tools may consist of interpretation, analysis, evaluation, inference, and explanation of the evidential, conceptual, methodological, criteriological, or contextual considerations.
Linda Elder (2007)—The Critical Thinking Community	Critical thinking is that mode of thinking—about any subject, content, or problem—in which the thinker improves the quality of his or her thinking by skillfully analyzing, assessing, and reconstructing it. Critical thinking is self-directed, self-disciplined, self-monitored, and self-corrective thinking. It presupposes assent to rigorous standards of excellence and mindful command of their use. It entails effective communication and problem-solving abilities, as well as a commitment to overcome our native egocentrism and sociocentrism.
National League for Nursing Accreditation Commission (NLNAC)	The deliberate nonlinear process of collecting, interpreting, analyzing, drawing conclusions about, presenting, and evaluating information that is both factually and belief based. This is demonstrated in nursing by clinical judgment, which includes ethical, diagnostic, and therapeutic dimensions and research (p. 8).
The American Association of Colleges of Nurses (AACN)	Critical thinking underlies independent and interdependent decision making. Critical thinking includes questioning, analysis, synthesis, interpretation, inference, inductive and deductive reasoning, intuition, application, and creativity (p. 9).

The combination of these definitions is used to identify the scope and key elements for critical thinking in many nursing programs. This allows programs to validate critical thinking in applying learned knowledge and skills to the identification of patient problems and performing appropriate nursing actions for promotion of positive patient outcomes. Critical thinking skills are cultivated in all aspects of nursing education using foundational liberal arts and science courses taken outside the nursing curriculum.

Critical Thinking: An Essential Component of Nursing Practice

Critical thinking is potentially the single most important factor that determines success or failure in nursing practice. Activities used by nurses in the workplace incorporate independent and group problem solving, resource allocation, integration of data and information using technology, and acquiring and evaluating numerous amounts of information. Success in using these activities requires that the nurse possess basic educational skills like reading and writing; personality attributes that promote personal interaction and trust, such as self-esteem, self-confidence, self-awareness of limitations; and thinking skills that include the ability to reason, generate ideas, and problem solve.

Critical thinking allows the nurse to examine current scenarios, analyze all relevant information, and make decisions based on the best course of action. This promotes competent care delivery. As nurses become more experienced, their ability to critically think is enhanced. This ability is described by Dr. Patricia Benner in her research and work describing five levels of expertise from novice to expert (see Table 2).

The length of time one is exposed to care activities promotes changes in skill level. Differences in levels of skills reflect changes in three aspects of skill performance. These include:

1. Moving from relying on context-free rules that are applied universally to using past concrete experiences to guide care actions.
2. Change from viewing situations as separate pieces to a holistic view and perspective of the whole.
3. Movement from a passive observer outside of the situations to an involved performer actively engaged and participating.

Critical thinking in nursing encourages the nurse to be "habitually inquisitive, well-informed, trustful of reason, open-minded, flexible, fair-minded in evaluation, honest in facing personal biases, prudent in making judgments, willing to reconsider, clear about issues, orderly in complex matters, diligent in seeking relevant information, reasonable in the selection of criteria, focused in inquiry, and persistent in seeking results which are as precise as the subject and the circumstances of inquiry permit" (Facione, 1990, p. 2). Critical thinking serves as a foundation for sound clinical

Table 2. Benner's Levels of Nursing Experience

Level of Experience	Descriptors
1. Novice	• Beginner with no experience.
	• Taught general rules to assist with performing tasks.
	• Rules are context-free and applied universally.
	• Rule-governed behavior is limited and inflexible.
2. Advanced Beginner	• Demonstrates acceptable (marginal) performance of tasks.
	• Has difficulty generating priorities and may view situations as having the same level of importance.
	• Has gained prior experience in real situations to recognize recurring meaningful components.
	• Principles are based on experiences and form a foundation to guide actions.
3. Competent	• Demonstrates competence in task performance with usually 2 to 3 years of experience.
	• Gains perspective from planning own actions based on conscious, abstract. and analytical thinking.
	• Thinks abstractly and efficiently organizes activities for simultaneous implementation.
4. Proficient	• Perceives and understands situations as part of a whole.
	• Uses holistic understanding to improve decision making.
	• Learns from prior experience what to expect in certain situations.
	• Uses prior experience to modify plans for situational management.
5. Expert	• Does not rely on principles, rules, or guidelines to determine actions.
	• Has an intuitive grasp of situations.
	• Performance is fluid and flexible.
	• Highly proficient and responds automatically.

Adapted from Benner, P. (1984). *From Novice to Expert: Excellence and Power in Clinical Nursing Practice.* Menlo Park: Addison-Wesley

judgment in the health care setting. These judgment decisions ultimately affect patient outcomes. There are cognitive skills and traits/dispositions of critical thinkers. These are identified in Table 3.

To see how you add up as a critical thinker, answer the questions in Table 4. Rate your use of each component as poor, good, or excellent. For those areas that you rate as poor, develop a plan to increase your proficiency and use of this component in your everyday life, which will transfer to nursing.

The key to developing critical thinking is continuous learning. Through the use of lifelong learning activities, you can increase your knowledge and improve the depth of your clinical judgment. A self-assessment is a good place to start the critical thinking process.

The Nursing Process

The nursing process is a mechanism used by nurses to critically solve problems in professional practice. This method of critical thinking uses a series of techniques to address an issue in patient management. This process is a cycle that moves fluidly from one step to the other (see Figure 1). Movement through the cycle allows for individualized care administration and consideration of varied alternatives for outcome generation by the experienced nurse. This dynamic, interactive process includes a

Table 3. Cognitive Skills and Traits/Dispositions of Critical Thinkers

Cognitive Skills	Traits/Dispositions
<ul><li>Interpretation—categorization, decoding significance, clarifying meaning</li><li>Analysis—examining ideas, detecting, and analyzing arguments</li><li>Evaluation—assessing claims and arguments</li><li>Inference—querying evidence, conjecturing alternatives, drawing conclusions</li><li>Explanation—stating results, justifying procedures, presenting arguments</li><li>Self-monitoring—self-examination and correction</li><li>Information seeking, Discriminating, Predicting, Applying Standards, Logical reasoning</li></ul>	<ul><li>Truth-seeking—courageous about asking questions, honest and objective in pursuing inquiry</li><li>Open-mindedness—sensitive to own bias, respect rights of others to hold differing opinions</li><li>Analyticity—alert to potentially problematic situations</li><li>Systematicity—organized, orderly, focused, diligent inquiry</li><li>Self-confidence—trust in own reasoning</li><li>Inquisitiveness—intellectual curiosity, values being well informed</li><li>Maturity—disposed to make reflective judgments</li><li>Reflection, Perseverance, Contextual perspective, Creativity, Flexibility, Intuition</li></ul>

From Scheffer, B. K., & Rubenfeld, M. G. (2000). A consensus statement on critical thinking in nursing. *Journal of Nursing Education, 39*(8), 352–359.

Table 4. Critical Thinking Self-Assessment

Component	Yes	Sometimes	No
I can work with change in a situation by making a logical plan for a successful outcome.			
I can tell the difference between fact and opinion when coming to a decision.			
I can evaluate evidence for use in making a decision.			
I recognize biases in myself and others.			
I value the opinion of others.			
I change my opinion when I find evidence that verifies that I am not correct.			
I recognize and can work within my own limitations.			
I am comfortable with the idea that there may be more than one answer or solution to a problem.			
I look at a situation from different directions or perspectives.			
I am organized and orderly in my approach to solving a problem.			
I use knowledge from previous situations in making decisions regarding current situations.			
I try to learn from my mistakes.			

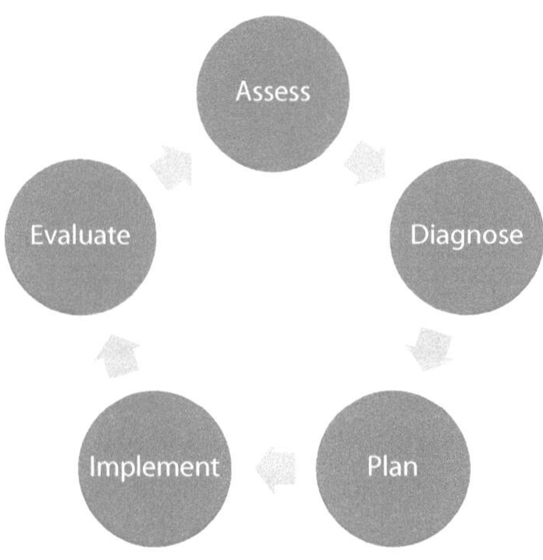

Figure 1. The Nursing Process

reciprocal interpersonal relationship between patient and nurse. The nurse often engages with one patient in numerous activities that are at various steps in the process simultaneously; for example, the nurse may be at the assessment step for a projected ambulation activity and at the step of implementation for a patient teaching activity. The nursing process is also flexible, and it can be used in any health care setting with patients of any age or developmental level.

Step 1: Assess the Patient

Assessment starts the process for responding to actual (what is happening now) or potential (what could happen) patient problems. It involves collecting information from the patient, family, or other individuals who may impact the patient's health status. Information is collected regarding immediate health issues, historical information regarding health issues, insurance status, and pharmacological history. Holistic information is retrieved from developmental, physiological, psychological, sociological, cultural, spiritual, and environmental perspectives. How this information is made a permanent part of the patient record will depend on the template and format (electronic versus hard copy) used by the organization.

Collecting Patient Data

Data is collected through interview (see Figure 2) and physical examination. The interview starts the process and sets the stage for the development of trust between the patient and nurse. Usually this is done face to face upon entry to a care setting. Occasionally, it may be done by phone or collected electronically. Even if other methods are used, a face-to-face validation session will occur between patient and nurse.

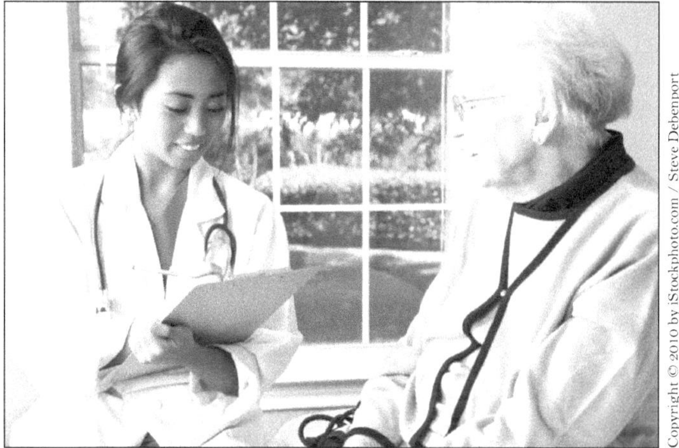

Figure 2. Interviewing starts the nursing process and lays the foundation for care delivery.

Interviewing is a vital skill in beginning a trusting relationship and collecting key information upon which to base future care activities. Some tips for conducting an interview that promotes a good outcome include:

- Clearly articulate the purpose of the interview and all questions.
- Choose an interview location that allows for comfort and privacy.
- Attempt to be on the same level as the patient (do not stand over the patient, as this may impede communication).
- Use various question types to encourage communication of information
- open questions that encourage verbalization (e.g., "What brought you to the clinic today?")
- closed questions that promote one- or two-word responses of factual information (e.g., "How old are you?")
- Do not combine multiple issues when asking questions (e.g., "Do you have heart disease, hypertension, or diabetes?")
- Do not use questions that may lead the patient to answer in a specific way (e.g., "You don't have any heart disease in your family, do you?"—gives the impression that heart disease is bad and may prompt the patient to answer no incorrectly).
- Listen attentively to responses.

Patient information may be organized as it is being collected since much of this information will be immediately placed on a hard copy form or input to a computerized template and made part of the permanent patient record.

Information is also retrieved by physical examination of the patient. Assessment techniques include inspection, palpation, percussion, and auscultation to obtain information that expands the base of patient data. This allows for investigation of body systems and functions to further validate other information collected from the patient or other source. This promotes movement to subsequent areas of the nursing process.

Types of Data

Two types of patient data are collected: subjective and objective. Subjective data is information supplied by the patient in the form of complaints and descriptions about their current health issue. This is what the patient says or actually tells you is wrong. Examples can include "I have a pain in my leg"; "My wrist hurts when I try to pick up something"; or "I have been vomiting since yesterday." It should be put in quotation marks since it is a quote of the actual words of the patient. The only source for this information is the patient.

Objective data are signs that can be observed, measured, and verified through the senses. It can be collected through observation or examination. This data can be retrieved through measurement techniques such as temperature, heart rate, respiration, and/ or blood pressure. Another term for this data is "signs." It is a sign of something that is going on with the patient. Examples of this type of data include red swollen joints, grimacing when a joint is moved, an open and bleeding wound, or a patient holding their stomach in pain.

These two types of data can be used to validate each other. They should have agreement between them. If a patient describes having a painful ankle after a fall (subjective data) and the ankle is swollen and shows evidence of bruising (objective data), these two pieces of information would be in agreement. If the patient complains of a painful ankle (subjective) and there is no sign of swelling or bruising (objective data), these two pieces of information would not be in agreement. Information that is not in agreement may identify problems that are not physiological but rather psychological in nature. Through the use of astute interviewing skills by the nurse, other problems may be identified that may need to be addressed.

Sources of Patient Data

Information may be obtained from three sources: primary, secondary, or tertiary. The primary data source is the patient and any information collected directly from this individual. Secondary sources include family, friends, or the nurse's own knowledge from prior interactions or observations. Tertiary sources are sources that compile or digest other sources, such as the patient's medical record. Since other health care providers are a source of synthesized information (e.g., they hold information from the patient's medical regimen, including laboratory data, prior medical information, intervention strategies, etc.), they too may be considered as tertiary sources.

Confidentiality of Patient Information

Information collected by nurses may include very personal and confidential types of data. It is important to maintain the strictest confidence for this information. Establishing a trusting relationship means that the nurse has a legal and ethical obligation to guard this information from inadvertent disclosure. It is important to remember that patient information is confidential and comes under the Health Insurance Portability and Accountability Act (HIPAA) ruling for disclosure on a need-to-know basis. This may be difficult when information is collected in partially open areas. Every effort must be made to prevent others from overhearing this information (e.g., lowering voices, closing doors, or pulling curtains to reduce vocalizations). Electronic information should not be accessed out of curiosity or personal interest. Electronic access or data retrieval is only accepted in an organization by health care providers who have direct care responsibilities for a patient. This means that no discussion of a patient should occur in the cafeteria or elevator. Even if no identifying information is disclosed it may not be difficult for others who work in an area to clearly identify an individual from the smallest piece of information. Information discussions between members of the health care team should also be done in an area that promotes privacy and eliminates the probability of inadvertent disclosure of information to another person.

<h1 style="text-align:center">Step 2: Formulate the Nursing Diagnosis</h1>

Based on information collected and organized in the assessment phase, a process of reasoning is used to identify problems and develop nursing diagnoses. Information should be organized into groups in order to facilitate analysis and identification of problems related to each specific group (see Figure 3). Systematic organization allows easy review, analysis, and identification of nursing diagnoses related to each body system (e.g., neurological system, cardiovascular system, gastrointestinal system, etc.).

Nursing diagnoses differ from medical diagnoses as nursing diagnoses focus on patient problems that nurses are capable of managing. A nursing diagnosis is a human response to "actual or potential health problems which nurses, by virtue of their education and experience are capable and licensed to treat" (Gordon, 1976, p. 1299). They may be related to the individual, family, or community. They focus on the human response and may address the patient's physical, sociocultural, psychological, and/or spiritual response to an illness or health problem. The nurse is responsible and accountable for outcomes of a nursing diagnosis. A medical diagnosis is specific and related to a pathological disease process. These are diagnoses that require medical or surgical intervention.

Nursing diagnoses are standardized by a professional organization known as NANDA International (NANDI-I) (formerly known as the North American Nursing Diagnosis Association) which is located at http://www.nanda.org. This organization facilitates development, refinement, dissemination, and the use of standard terminology for nursing diagnoses. They promote research to establish evidence-based nursing diagnoses for use in nursing practice in order to identify interventions and outcomes that contribute to safe clinical decisions. They continue to develop and refine nursing diagnoses with input from nurses worldwide.

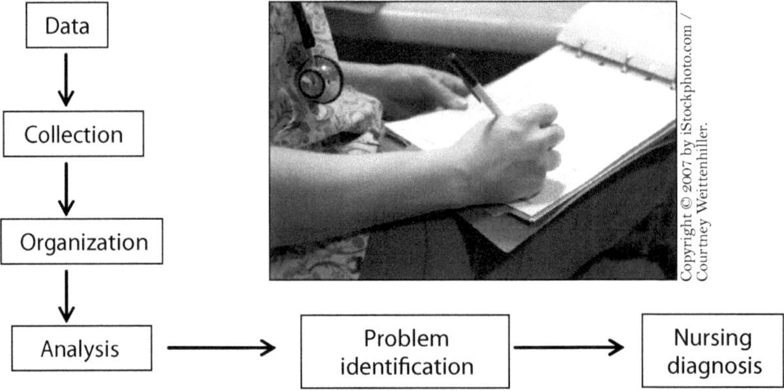

Figure 3. Process of Nursing Diagnosis Formulation

Many nursing programs use nursing diagnoses in identification and development of care plans or plans for care for patient intervention. These can be developed with help from the list of NANDA-approved nursing diagnoses. The initial part of the nursing diagnosis is the label, which is the concise term or phrase that names the specific diagnosis from the NANDA list. This information is followed consecutively by the: Definition or term/phrase that delineates meaning and differentiates it from other similar diagnoses, defining characteristics that are observable components such as signs and symptoms, risk factors that increase vulnerability to an unhealthy event, and related factors that precede, are associated with, or relate to the diagnosis. An example of a nursing diagnosis would be:

A format for writing nursing diagnoses uses the **PES** format. This includes a **P**roblem, **E**tiology, and **S**igns and symptoms component (see Figure 4).

The nursing diagnosis would be constructed based on this format (see Figure 5):

The nursing diagnosis in Figure 5 would be written out as "Imbalanced nutrition, less than body requirements related to inadequate daily caloric intake AEB loss of 30 pounds in six months." All nursing diagnoses would follow this construction format. Now use the activity in Table 5 to test your knowledge of nursing versus medical diagnoses. Select the correct category for each diagnosis in the table. The correct answers can be found at the end of the chapter.

Following identification of nursing diagnoses, it is important to prioritize these based on patient safety and harm that may occur. Maslow's hierarchy of needs may also be used to prioritize these (see Figure 6). Lower needs are more fundamental and needed for survival (physiological and safety). Nursing diagnoses that fit into these two categories should be addressed first and in the order presented in the diagram, with physiological needs taking priority over safety needs.

A nursing diagnosis that deals with a situation that threatens a physiological need would be addressed first by the nurse. This would mean that a nursing diagnosis of "ineffective airway clearance" would be dealt with before "sleep pattern disturbance"

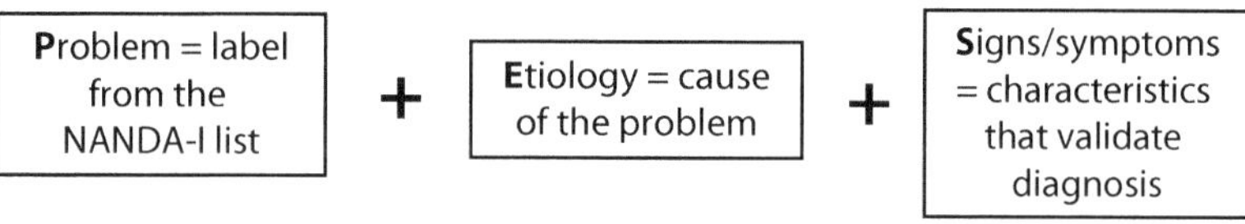

Figure 4. Format for writing nursing diagnosis statement

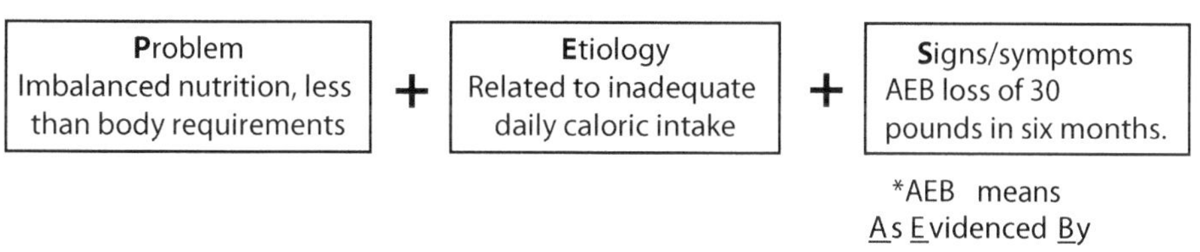

Figure 5. Nursing diagnosis construction

Table 5. Activity to Identify Nursing versus Medical Diagnoses*

Diagnoses	Nursing Diagnosis	Medical Diagnosis
1. Ineffective airway clearance		
2. Asthma		
3. Hypertension		
4. Activity intolerance		
5. Sleep pattern disturbance		
6. Diabetes		
7. Fluid volume excess		
8. Congestive heart failure		
9. Pain, acute		
10. Skin integrity, impaired		

*Correct answers at end of chapter.

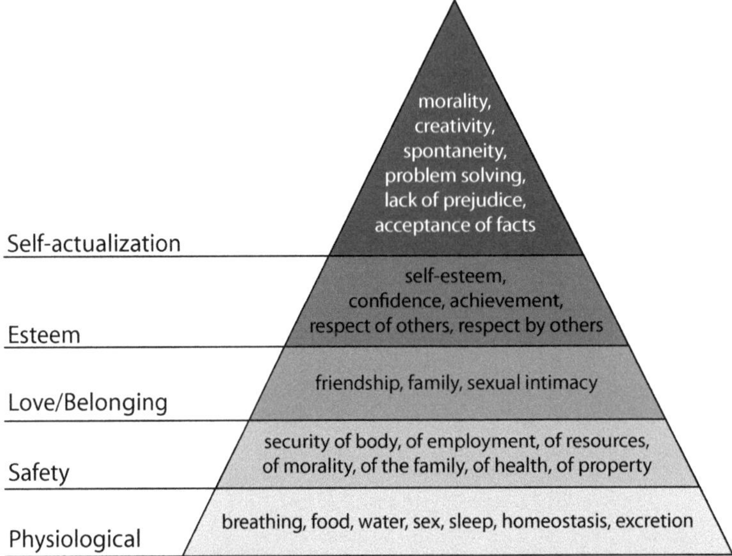

"Maslow's Hierarchy of Needs" © Factoryjoe, (CC BY-SA 3.0) at: http://en.wikipedia.org/wiki/File:Maslow%27s_Hierarchy_of_Needs.svg.

Figure 6. Maslow's Hierarchy of Needs

from Table 5. When possible, nurses should involve patients in their care by working with them to identify and prioritize nursing diagnoses. They can assist in identifying those diagnoses that do not relate to life-threatening situations, but rather to feelings of self-worth and knowledge on a specific topic. This can serve to educate the patient and promote self-care and ownership in personal care outcomes.

Step 3: Plan for Provision of Patient Care

The third step in the nursing process is planning for patient care. At this step, problems that have been prioritized are taken further and worked through stages needed to accomplish a successful outcome. All needs cannot be addressed simultaneously. The first stage is to identify which needs are immediate and which ones can be delayed. Those needs requiring immediate attention, such as those that are life-threatening, are addressed first. In the second stage, goals or outcome statements for planning nursing actions will need to be established. Patient goals may be long term or short term. Long-term goals are those that require weeks to months to achieve, whereas short-term goals can be achieved in hours or days. It is good to have both types of goals. Long-term goals keep the patient working to achieve maximum potential. Short-term goals give a sense of accomplishment and promote self-esteem. These can keep patient momentum for goals that do not show change over several days or weeks. The third stage is to determine interventions. These need to be specific and directed toward realistic outcomes for the patient. Interventions can range from safety measures (e.g., bed side rails up and bed in low position at all times) to activities that promote sleep and rest (e.g., promote quiet atmosphere by closing room door and coordinating disruptive activities). In selecting appropriate interventions, it is important to remember that they must be:

- Safe for intervention.
- Appropriate for the patient's age and overall health.
- Consistent with the patient's values, beliefs, and culture.
- Compatible with collaborative therapies of other health care professionals.
- Within established Standards of Nursing Care.
- Based on knowledge and experience of the nurse.
- Evidence based.

Planning should be focused to meet one of the three types of planning: initial planning, ongoing planning, and discharge planning. These are not mutually exclusive, but can occur simultaneously. Initial planning is important to retrieve historical information and address immediate needs (e.g., postsurgical patient admission). Ongoing planning is what occurs throughout the interactive nurse-patient period of involvement over a given period of time (e.g., shift of work). This is necessary to determine appropriate care necessary to address patient care. Discharge planning is necessary to promote self-care and prepare the individual to address issues related to health following discharge from the facility. This should start on admission in order to allow time for learning to occur. Continuous feedback promotes learning and builds confidence in performing self-care activities.

Nursing interventions can be independent, dependent, or collaborative. Independent interventions are those that can be initiated by a nurse, such as physical care and ongoing assessment of the patient. Dependent interventions are those that are carried out under the specific order of a physician, for instance, administration of medication or special dressing management postsurgical intervention. Collaborative interventions are actions that nurses carry out in a cooperative manner with other health professionals, such as managing the pulmonary status of a patient in collaboration with the respiratory therapist.

Step 4: Implement Plan of Care

Implementation of nursing actions identified in the plan is the fourth step in the nursing process. This is where the plan is actually put into action through implementation of nursing activities. Before the plan is implemented, it is important to (a) review and validate the plan in order to make any modifications that may be required, since the plan may be written hours or days before it is actually implemented; (b) assess and correlate current level of knowledge and skills compared to actual knowledge and skills needed to implement the plan and request assistance as needed; (c) prepare the patient for nursing actions and expectations; and (d) prepare the environment for implementation activities.

These activities should be nursing focused and patient centered. Care activities should be individualized to meet current health care needs. Activities should be focused toward successful achievement of goals and objectives. Competent, safe nursing interactions will be needed to address all needs identified in the plan. Care activities should be carried out efficiently in order to conserve energy and promote healing for the patient. As activities are implemented, the nurse should continue to evaluate the patient response in order to make any adjustments to the plan during care activities. Other activities may also alter the patient care plan. For example, a nursing intervention may be identified that states the patient is to be ambulated for 30 minutes based on a predetermined schedule but following an interventional procedure (e.g., lumbar puncture, also called a spinal tap), this activity may need to be altered to allow for a restricted reclining position for a designated period of time based on physician orders. Additional measures may need to be implemented based on the patient's physical condition prior to the procedure, which were not in the original plan for the patient. These may include increased rest for 24 hours and reduction of activities, including ambulation and exercise, for a period of time.

This phase also requires documentation of activities performed and the patient's response. Documentation should be sequential based on time of activity implementation. Do not chart activities done at 2 pm before activities completed at 12:30 pm. It is good to chart as close to an activity as possible in order to accurately reflect all parts of the activity—nursing activity and patient response. Some organizations have electronic charting, which allows for almost immediate documentation since computer stations are in the patient room, on mobile carts, or centrally located close to patient care rooms. Charting is a legal responsibility of the nurse and is a part of the permanent patient record.

Step 5: Evaluate Outcome

The fifth step in the nursing process is evaluation. At this time, the nurse systematically compares the patient's health status against identified goals and expected outcomes. This step involves the nurse, patient, and other members of the health care team. At this step the patient status, progress toward goal, and outcome achievement and effectiveness of nursing strategies are evaluated.

Using the nursing diagnosis of "Fluid volume deficit related to fluid loss from vomiting and diarrhea AEB signs of dehydration and loss of 10 pounds over seven days," the expected outcome may state: The patient will maintain normal fluid balance and increased weight by discharge AEB:

- Increased body weight
- Normal skin turgor (elasticity of the skin)
- Moist mucous membranes
- Stable vital signs (blood pressure, heart rate, and respiratory rate) while supine, sitting, and standing
- No episodes of vomiting or diarrhea.

Evaluation would validate that the patient has gained three pounds since admission and has normal elastic skin with moist and pink mucous membranes. Vital signs are stable in all positions with no significant changes and there have been no episodes of vomiting or diarrhea in 72 hours. In this situation, the goal was met. There may be two other outcomes for patients related to goal achievement. Goals may be partially met or not met. For goals that are achieved, the patient's problem is resolved or a potential problem prevented. If the goal was achieved but the patient's problem persists, there may have been a mismatch between the stated goal and the patient's current condition. This will require revision of the care plan. Regardless of the outcome, charting should occur. For goals that are not met or partially met, there should be a reassessment of the situation, with revisions of the plan for patient care. Evaluation should identify why goals were partially achieved or not achieved. Some reasons might include:

- There was a mismatch between the client's capabilities and the goal, making the goal unrealistic.
- The nursing diagnosis was not accurate and did not correctly reflect the actual or potential problem.
- Nursing actions did not match the goal or did not achieve a level sufficient to address the goal.
- Medical intervention and/or orders changed, affecting nursing and patient priorities.
- The patient's condition changed, which required a change in health care interventions from the interdisciplinary team, including nursing.
- The patient and/or family decided to alter the plan due to a change in the direction of desired care (e.g., change in the patient's advanced directive for health care).

Evaluation is part of this continuous process for nursing and allows for measurement of quality, appropriateness, and effectiveness of care. Actual care delivered should correlate to the plan of care and promote achievement of collaborative goals.

The nursing process is a problem-solving technique that requires practice, the same as any other skill in nursing. The process provides a framework for responsible and accountable nursing care. Using this process in a nonlinear format may promote clinical reasoning in patient management. This is done more efficiently by the experienced nurse, who does not visualize the process as moving from one step to the next and only in a forward direction but moves between the steps repeating and revising them as necessary prior to arriving at a solution.

Clinical reasoning is a critical skill that allows the nurse to formulate wise decisions. This thinking process promotes the performance of the best-judged action in a specific situation. It is a combination of several attributes (see Figure 7) that result from formal and informal thinking processes. It is dynamic and allows the nurse to retrieve information, analyze it for relevance, and elect to use or discard the information or reserve it for later use in the process. Information continuously goes through this process, integrating organizational policies, level of patient care needed, collaborative level required for implementation, and level of experience to carry out needed interventions.

Critical thinking and clinical reasoning are closely aligned in that they both are techniques used for problem solving. Fonteyn's (1991) definition of clinical reasoning addressed it as a cognitive process that nurses use during review and analysis of patient information when planning care activities to promote positive patient outcomes. Clinical reasoning is established as the nurse gains knowledge and expertise. It has as its primary objective to promote decisions that resolve problems. These decisions are developed by the experienced nurse by using predictive reasoning based on knowledge and prior exposure to the situation with other patients, backward reasoning by searching for previous data that gives an explanation for a clinical suspicion, and forward reasoning, which incorporates new data into the developed plan of care in an effort to make clinical decisions for the best patient outcome.

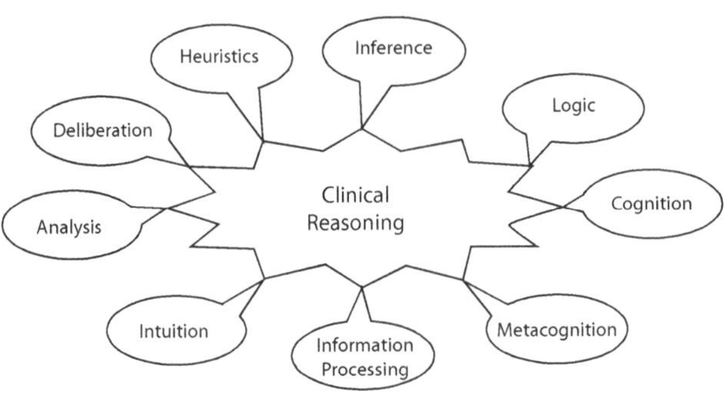

Adapted from Simmons, B. (2010). Clinical reasoning: Concept analysis. *Journal of Advanced Nursing, 66*(5), 1151–1158.

Figure 7. Attributes of Clinical Reasoning

Clinical reasoning is dependent on the nurse collecting critical information. These are identified by Levett-Jones, et al. (2010) as the five rights of clinical reasoning:

1. The right cues.
2. The right action.
3. The right patient.
4. The right time.
5. The right reason.

Use of the five rights is just one strategy the nurse can use to promote clinical reasoning in developing a decision for patient management. Critical inquiry is also a process of examining existing assumptions, knowledge, and questions. The nurse can then move to gaining and creating new information needed to address a patient care issue. This leads to gaining new perspectives, critical analysis, sharing what was learned, action, and reflection. This process allows the nurse to identify a problem, propose a solution, locate evidence for validation (for or against proposed solutions), and evaluate solutions based on the evidence. The nurse examines and challenges current situations used for patient management and identifies potential evidence-based solutions.

Summary

There is no one technique or strategy used by nurses in clinical settings to arrive at solutions for clinical problems. The nurse may use several strategies for development of clinical expertise and promotion of problem-solving techniques that promote the best patient outcome. Mind actions may occur in various combinations to achieve an outcome. Clinical reasoning and critical inquiry are but two strategies that incorporate recognition of a situation that needs intervention, reflection on known information to make a wise decision, interpretation of that information, and action or movement toward an outcome. It is important for the nurse to know how to incorporate these methods into "thinking on your feet" as they move from situation to situation.

References

Alfaro-LeFevre, R. (2004). *Critical Thinking and Clinical Judgment: A Practical Approach.* (3rd ed.). Philadelphia: W. B. Saunders.

American Philosophical Association. (1990). Critical thinking: A statement of expert consensus for purposes of educational assessment and instruction. ERIC document, ED 315–423.

Benner, P. (1984). *From Novice to Expert.* Menlo Park, CA: Addison-Wesley.

Elder, L. (2007). Our concept of critical thinking: A definition. Retrieved from http://www.criticalthinking.org/page.cfm?PageID=411&CategoryID=51

Facione, P. A. (1990). *Critical Thinking: A Statement of Expert Consensus for Purpose of Educational Assessment and Instruction, Executive Summary, "The Delphi Report."* Millbrae, CA: California Academic Press.

Fonteyn, M. (1991). A descriptive analysis of expert critical care nurses' clinical reasoning. Doctoral Dissertation. University of Texas, Austin, TX.

Fonteyn, M., & Fisher, A. (1995). An innovative methodological approach for examining nurses' heuristic use in clinical practice. *Journal of Scholarly Inquiry*, 9, 263–276.

Gordon, M. (1987). *Nursing Diagnosis: Process and Application.* 2nd ed. New York: McGraw-Hill.

Institute of Medicine. (2004). Keeping patients safe: Transforming the work environment of nurses. Executive Summary, 2. Retrieved March 30, 2004 from http://books.nap.edu/books/030909679/html/index.html

Jennings, L. B., & Potter-Smith, C. (2002). Examining the role of critical inquiry for transformative practices: Two joint cases of multicultural teacher education. *Teachers College Record*, 104(3), 456–481.

Levett-Jones, T., Hoffman, K., Dempsey, J., Yeun-Sim Jeong, S., Noble, D., Norton, C. A., Rouche, J., & Hickey, N. (2010). The "five rights" of clinical reasoning: An educational model to enhance nursing students' ability to identify and manage clinically "at risk" patients. *Nurse Education Today*, 30(6), 515–520.

Locsin, R. C. (2001). The dilemma of decision-making: Processing thinking critical to nursing. *Holistic Nursing Practice*, 15(3), 1–3.

National League for Nursing Accreditation Commission (NLNAC) (2002). Accreditation manual. Retrieved from http://www.nlnac.org .

Scheffer, B. K., & Rubenfeld, M. G. (2000). A consensus statement on critical thinking in nursing. *Journal of Nursing Education*, 39(8), 352–359.

Simmons, B. (2010). Clinical reasoning: Concept analysis. *Journal of Advanced Nursing*, 66(5), 1151–1158. doi:10.1111/j.1365-2648.2010.05262.x.

Table 5. Activity to Identify Nursing versus Nursing Diagnoses (correct responses)

Diagnoses	Nursing Diagnosis	Medical Diagnosis
1. Ineffective airway clearance	X	
2. Asthma		
3. Hypertension		X
4. Activity intolerance	X	X
5. Sleep pattern disturbance	X	
6. Diabetes		X
7. Fluid volume excess	X	
8. Congestive heart failure		X
9. Pain, acute	X	
10. Skin integrity, impaired	X	

Chapter 7: Ethical Aspects of Nursing

Ethics is a very complex issue and may have no clear right or wrong answers based on the scenario. Ethical dilemmas are created by societal changes, technological advances, and changes in laws, regulations, and reimbursement. Decisions are further complicated by conflicts in patient's wishes and family member desires. Nurses face these situations daily as they strive to balance patient advocacy, moral philosophies, and personal values. These conflicts can cause psychological distress to the nurse. It is important for the nurse to be knowledgeable about how to blend all of these issues into a decision that represents balance.

Ethics and Morals

Nursing literature interchanges the terms ethics and morals but they are not the same. Morals are principles or standards of conduct regarding behaviors or beliefs that are acceptable or not regarding a situation. These established rules of conduct are used in situations where "right and wrong" decisions are needed relative to what is done. An individual's personal standards may serve as an individual thermometer for these decisions. The basis of these decisions is from societal attitudes and norms that are conveyed through customs, tradition, and religion. Recognition with individual reference groups may also be used. These reference groups may be based on age, gender, profession, and ethnicity, among others. Group references may overlap and promote stability in making a decision or cause an imbalance if references do not match on a specific situation. Morals may be learned through exposure to situations that require choices. Selection of the right choices may be facilitated through exposure to parental controls, formal education of policing laws, and culture. Peer and societal expectations as well as personal values also affect choices regarding moral issues.

Ethics are moral principles that govern an individual or group's behavior. It involves critical analysis of a situation to identify what should be done based on habits or customs. This requires consideration of all possible known actions in order to make the best ethical decision in a given situation. Codes of behavior may also be used to guide these decisions. In nursing, this is the American Nurses Association's (ANA) Code of Ethics for Nurses (see Box 1).

The International Council of Nurses (ICN) also developed a Code of Ethics for Nurses in 1953. The ICN is an organization that includes more than 130 national nursing associations and represents more than 13 million nurses worldwide. Its goals are to shape nursing into a global collective, to advance the profession of nursing worldwide, and to influence health policy on a worldwide scale.

The organization has continued to revise the ICN Code with updates based on the world's ever evolving and changing social perspectives which affect nursing's professional focus in response to these situations (e.g., telehealth, telenursing). The most recent revision was in 2005. The *ICN Code of Ethics for Nurses* has four principal elements which include (a) a nurse's responsibility to provide care to all individuals; (b) a requirement for personal responsibility and accountability to maintain competence in practice; (c) assuming a key role in identifying and implementing acceptable standards of clinical nursing in all areas which include practice, management, research and education; and (d) sustaining a supportive relationship with peers and colleagues.

Box 1. Code of Ethics for Nurses

Provision 1. The nurse, in all professional relationships, practices with compassion and respect for the inherent dignity, worth, and uniqueness of every individual, unrestricted by considerations of social considerations of social or economic status, personal attributes, or the nature of health problems.

Provision 2. The nurse's primary commitment is to the patient, whether an individual, family, group or community.

Provision 3. The nurse promotes, advocates for, and strives to protect the health, safety, and rights of the patient.

Provision 4. The nurse is responsible and accountable for individual nursing practice and determines the appropriate delegation of tasks consistent with the nurse's obligation to provide optimum patient care.

Provision 5. The nurse owes the same duties to self as to others, including the responsibility to preserve integrity and safety, maintain competence, and to continue personal and professional growth.

Provision 6. The nurse participates in establishing, maintaining, and improving health care environments and conditions of employment conducive to the provision of quality health care and consistent with the values of the profession through individual and collection action.

Provision 7. The nurse participates in the advancement of the profession through contributions to practice, education, administration, and knowledge development.

Provision 8. The nurse collaborates with other health professionals and the public in promoting community, national and international efforts to meet health needs.

Provision 9. The profession of nursing, as represented by associations and their members, is responsible for articulating nursing values, for maintaining the integrity of the profession and its practice, and for shaping social policy.

"Code of Ethics for Nurses with Interpretative Statements," Retrieved from www.nursingworld.org/Main-MenuCategories/EthicsStandards/CodeofEthicsforNurses/Code-of-Ethics.aspx. Copyright © by American Nurses Association. Reprinted with permission.

Ethical dilemmas are complex situations that result from a debate between two moral principles. In this situation, both sides have responses that may be reasonable to consider. Technological advances can be one source of these dilemmas. Advances have served to prolong life for individuals who, prior to technology, would not have survived (see Figure 1).

Devices such as ventilators for respiratory support and left ventricular assist devices to promote the workings of a defective heart may prolong the life of individuals who have no identifiable brain activity as evaluated by physical assessment or machine (an electroencephalogram can be used to detect brain wave activity). The mismatch of these signs of life and death generate questions related to quality of life and patient rights. Nurses must use ethics on a daily basis to arrive at decisions and ways to manage these patient care situations.

Basic Ethical Principles

Autonomy

Autonomy is the principle that states individuals have the right to make their own decisions and subsequently control their own lives. This principle is generally valued by individuals. It is often correlated to the concepts of "being my own person" and "shaping my own life." For patients, this principle focuses on situations where decisions are required for health care interventions. It is important that patients be offered options and allowed to make voluntary choices about these potentially life-changing decisions.

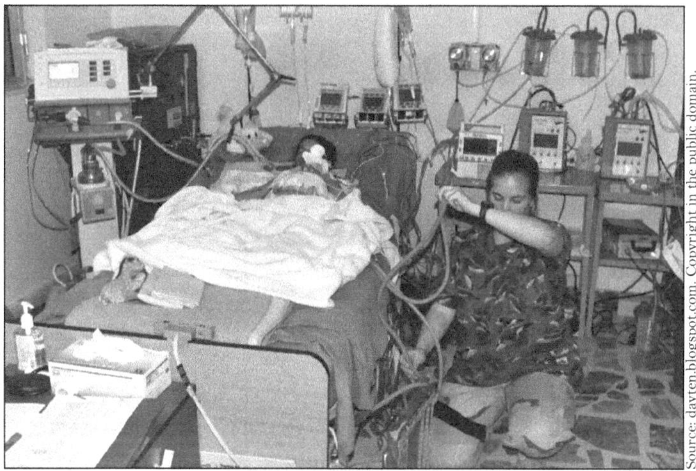

Figure 1. Technology in Patient Care

Autonomy is the ability of self-determination and is the moral foundation for informed consent. The patient's choice must be made without coercion or undue influence. This includes not using techniques such as gaining the assistance of outside influences to convince the patient, applying consequences, or coaxing. Respect for a patient's autonomy acknowledges their right to: hold views, make choices, and take actions based on personal values and beliefs. Each person is unique and deserves to have their life experiences respected because only they are aware of emotions, motivations, and physiological issues that govern their decisions. This requires that the health care professional respect the individual and their decisions. It is important that the individual is identified as old enough and competent to make these decisions. This means that they have the ability to make decisions regarding their own care and treatment based on information obtained from health care professionals, as well as refuse treatment regardless of the opinions of the care provider.

A situation that challenges autonomy is one that involves compulsory or forced treatment. This can result in a battle of wills between the patient ,who is determined to maintain autonomy, and the care provider, who is determined to treat the patient's illness. For example, a geriatric patient who is alert and oriented but in poor health and significant pain refuses to eat or drink. There is an alternative health care therapy called nasogastric tube feeding. In this method of feeding, a tube is inserted through the nose (usually) directly into the stomach in order to give the patient nutritional substances. But this procedure is considered invasive, requires collaborative management (e.g., medical, nursing, and nutritionist), and can be associated with complications. As with many ethical situations, there are several ethical principles involved in this scenario. Not only is autonomy an issue to be considered, but so is beneficence, nonmaleficence, and justice. These are explained below. Think of this scenario as you explore these ethical principles.

Beneficence

The principle of beneficence is one that is fundamental to nursing. When asked, many nursing students and professionals would say they desired to be a nurse in an effort "to help people." This directly reflects the health care professional's responsibility to contribute to the welfare of the patient. It means to do good, be proactive in helping others, and not engaging in activities that risk harming other persons. It requires that benefits and risks are balanced for the patient. Beneficence is the basis of the intent to work for the best interest of the patient. It is patient-centered and draws on care provider knowledge.

Questions arise from definitions of the term "good." When considering a definition for "good," it is important to consider the following questions:

- Who defines what is "good" for a patient?
- Is all life "good?"
- How does quality of life fit into what is "good" for a patient?

- Can a "good" death be better than a not-so-"good" life for patients with terminal illnesses?

Answers to these questions are not the same for all patients. Many things may affect the patient's answers, including personal importance of their place in society, feelings of obligation to family and friends, and perceived burden on others (physiological, psychological, emotional, and financial).

Nonmaleficence

Nonmaleficence is the principle that requires that health care providers do no harm. It reflects both the idea of not inflicting intentional harm and not engaging in activities or actions that risk harm to others. In health care, nonmaleficence includes avoiding negligent and harmful care. If, as the nurse, you fail to turn a patient every two hours and take precautions to prevent skin breakdown and the patient develops a decubitus ulcer, this would be a principle violation. This is because not turning the patient and taking precautions to prevent skin breakdown is negligent care, and as a result the patient was harmed by developing a decubitus ulcer. This situation is very clear in its violation, but often this is not the case. Some treatments cause temporary "harm" in an effort to give the possibility of a better life. This is the case with cancer treatment, which can include chemotherapy and radiation therapy. Some potential side effects include anemia (reduced red blood cells), appetite changes, bleeding problems, hair loss, fatigue (feeling tired), memory loss, mouth and throat changes that can affect the ability to eat, nausea and vomiting, pain, skin and nail changes, swelling (fluid retention), and urination changes. These can cause significant discomfort throughout the process of cancer treatment. The end result of this treatment may be a partial or complete remission. Partial remission would mean that a large percent of the signs and symptoms of cancer were gone but some still remain. Total remission would mean that there are no signs or symptoms of cancer. When caring for a patient experiencing these types of symptoms, it is difficult to view the treatment as not causing harm. It is important to remember that treatment was a decision made by the patient. The intent of the treatment is not to cause harm but rather as a potential to improve quality and length of life.

Fidelity

The ethical principle of fidelity is the obligation to be loyal, faithful, and to honor commitments. Patients should be able to trust their health care provider and have faith in the therapeutic relationship. It is important for health care team members to be faithful or loyal to agreements and responsibilities as part of their professional foundation. Not adhering to these important actions could threaten the therapeutic relationship between patient and care provider.

Fidelity supports the concept of accountability. Patients expect nurses to maintain fidelity when managing their care. This is reinforced by the organization when the nurse reports to duty. Patient assignments are made that identify nurse-patient care responsibility. The nurse is given a report on each patient to promote continuity of care, and the nurse accepts responsibility for the delivery of safe, professional care for a designated period of time. Throughout this time period, the nurse is accountable for delivery of care that complies with the ANA Code of Ethics and is within the scope of state nursing practice. Organizational policies and procedures also serve as a foundation for fidelity. Just as with other ethical principles, it is important to identify circumstances that would affect fidelity and its consequences.

Justice

Justice is the principle that states there should be social distribution of benefits and burdens. This means that decisions should be fair for all people. Everyone should be treated equally regardless of race, sex, religious beliefs, or life status (e.g., marital status, medical diagnosis, economic level, etc.). This principle underlies the first statement in the American Nurses Association (ANA) Code of Ethics, which states "The nurse in all professional relationships practices with compassion and respect for the inherent dignity, worth, and the uniqueness of every individual unrestricted by considerations of social or economic status, personal attributes, or the nature of health problems" (American Nurses Association, 2001). Justice is the promotion of equity or fairness in all nursing situations. This means that allocation of resources for nursing is done fairly; that would require nurses to engage in standards or criteria for ensuring equity for a staffing mix that addresses the needs of patients. It is also used by nurses when managing patient situations. Patients who are in need of immediate treatment are addressed first for care (e.g., responding to a bed alarm which would signal to the nurse that a patient on fall alert needs attention).

Another principle has its basis in justice. It is called distributive justice, which addresses the allocation of benefits. This expands on the justice principle by including a clause that defines justice as equal rights for everyone and the greatest benefit is to be given to the least advantaged persons or individuals with the greatest need. Evidence of this can be seen on the medical surgical unit where patients who are in pain have their needs addressed before a patient who is inquiring about discharge information.

Veracity

Veracity is the principle of truth telling. It is grounded in respect for persons and autonomy. This principle requires that the health care provider give the patient information necessary to make a rational decision based on available choices. The information delivered needs to be clear, internally consistent, coherent, comprehensive, and simple. Truth telling can be violated by health care providers if they (a) do not tell the truth or deliberately give the patient erroneous information; or (b) withhold information by omission or by deliberately using jargon that the patient cannot understand.

Informed consent is a significant part of this principle. Patients and families rely on information from caregivers in order to make informed choices regarding their health care. They expect to be told the truth even if it is to disclose a care provider error. Truth telling is expected regarding all forms of care activities.

Caregivers should be honest in their dealings with all individuals in addition to patients and their families. Truthfulness is expected in all patient and community interactions and activities. They should be honest in all forms of documentation, review of peers for professional activities, compliance with standards of care and organizational policies and procedures, communications and transactions with community individuals, and regulatory reporting to name a few.

Ethical Theories

Deontology

Deontology is a duty-based theory with a central moral concept of duty. It holds that some feature of an act, other than consequences, makes it right or wrong. Actions are based on a duty to perform certain activities. According to this theory, the most important aspects of our lives are governed by certain unbreakable moral rules. These rules may not be broken even if breaking them would improve the outcome. Using this theory means that ethical decision making is based on rules and principles regardless of the consequences.

The ethical theory of deontology focuses on what is right. These rights are governed by set rules that cannot be changed regardless of the consequences, even in health care situations. Using this theory results in predictable decisions because decisions are based on the individual's set duties and not the patient consequences or outcome. This is an example of a non-consequentialist theory, which means that it is based on something other than the rightness or wrongness of the consequences. This type of theory judges rightness and wrongness based on properties fundamental to the action, not the consequences.

The theory contends that individuals have a duty to do certain things and not do certain things. Based on this theory, one would never tell a lie regardless of the consequences of this action. An example would be a patient who requested that their family members not be told their cancer diagnosis. Based on deontological theory, if the patient's family asked, the caregiver would be required to tell a truth and some information even against the wishes of the patient. They would be required to respond in a manner that would not violate confidentiality. To tell the truth under any circumstances could be a significant constraint for this theory. The constraints caused by this theory are freely accepted by individuals who are bound to this theory and using this theory requires looking at the act itself, not the consequences.

Virtue Ethics

Virtue ethics identifies that an individual does the right thing knowingly and willfully. It does not take into account the reason for the action, but instead emphasizes the importance of personality traits in the response. This ethical theory can be found in the works of Plato and Aristotle. These Greek philosophers identified that virtue ethics was a collection of normative ethical philosophies which emphasized "being" rather than "doing." To them, moral virtues represented excellence of character and were displayed in characteristics such as courage, temperance, or excellence. Aristotle identified that virtues of character were acquired by practicing them and not just one exposure or situation. These take time to develop and internalize. According to Aristotle (c. 384 BC), the virtue of honesty could not be developed by performing one honest act. One act alone did not represent internalization of the virtue. Plato (c. 427 BC) identified that virtue was based on knowledge or wisdom. They both focused their questions of character around what type of person an individual should be.

Virtue ethics de-emphasizes rules, consequences, and specific acts and places the focus on the kind of person who is acting. It is not necessarily based on a right intention or whether a specific rule is followed, but rather on whether the person is expressing good character or not. This theory sees a person as the total sum of their virtues or character traits. These traits can range on a continuum from good to bad and are deeply entrenched in their person. Some character traits include being attentive, confident, cooperative, efficient, honest, polite, reliable, thoughtful, and trustworthy, among many others. Individuals develop character traits by habits of perception, motivation, and action. As a result, the individual who practices this ethical theory will act in a good way, not because of principle or duty, but rather because they are good.

Virtue ethics is used in one's personal and professional dealings with individuals. As an internalized part of the person, no distinction is made between personal and professional use of the virtue. Responding in such a way to take virtue ethics into consideration does not guarantee that an individual will engage in the correct behavior, but it does predispose them to the correct action.

Principlism

Principlism is a system of ethics that uses principles in place of theory and moral rules and ideals in addressing ethical situations. It is based on four ethical principles. These are autonomy (free will), beneficence (to do good), nonmaleficence (to do no harm), and justice (the social distribution of benefits and burdens). The four-principles approach of principlism is a generalist approach to addressing different ethical situations. Individuals who are proponents of principlism state that these four moral principles are evident in decisions of the past and are compatible with many intellectual individuals, religions, and cultural beliefs. This makes principlism a unified moral approach, where each principle assists in arriving at an ethical decision. The goal is to balance each principle, giving importance to each but not ranking them, as there is no intrinsic priority for these principles.. This allows each one to be used as an attribute to unify the decision-making process when dealing with ethical situations. This does not mean that one principle may not be more influential than the other in a given situation. Awareness of this change in balance allows the principlism user to work toward balance. This allows for the decision maker to get maximum benefit from each principle.

The four principles of autonomy, beneficence, nonmaleficence, and justice are role-specific duties that are always in effect when administering care. There can be a dilemma in using this system of ethics for the caregiver. For example, if a patient desires to discontinue taking a medication needed for health care management, the nurse may feel obligated to respect the patient's autonomy but compelled to promote patient wellness, which is the ethical role of beneficence (to do good). It is important for the principlism user to be aware of potential balance conflicts in using this system in managing ethical situations.

Consequentialism

In consequentialism, an action is right if it promotes the best consequences. This theory is result based and focuses on the right act. An act is better or more right if it produces more good consequences. This means that an ethical decision would be based on which act resulted in the best consequences for the patient. In consequentialism, an action should be chosen that maximizes good consequences. This theory is designed to maximize the good for a given situation. Based on consequentialism, lying would be wrong because it usually produces bad consequences. Utilitarianism is one form of consequentialism.

Utilitarianism

Utilitarianism looks at right and wrong from the perspective of promoting the greatest good for the greatest number of individuals. It seeks an answer to an ethical situation through the perspective of an answer to the question—What is the greatest good for the greatest number of people? In addition to this question, there is the premise of increasing human well-being or welfare, which is called "utility," the derivative term for the theory. In this theory, well-being for humans consists of pleasure.

Utilitarianism focuses on outcomes and not intentions for that outcome. This theory promotes no independent sense of right and wrong. According to Pollock (2004), good for many individuals outweighs a negative situation for one individual. This is very evident in disaster management. In a situation where hundreds of individuals are injured, some of them critically, time distribution for care management would be focused on helping as many individuals as possible instead of focusing numerous hours on the treatment of one person. Decision actions are judged and evaluated based on the achieved goal or outcome, which should result in a general good for the majority of individuals. This is also used by health care programs and other organizations in deciding the distribution of health care dollars. With limited monies available to a program or organization, they could use this theory to make a decision aimed at spending these dollars on immunizations for numerous individuals in the community as opposed to paying for a liver transplant for one individual. What makes this action right is the fact that it produced the best consequences.

Ethical Dilemmas

An ethical dilemma is a moral problem or situation that can have two or more mutually exclusive—yet morally correct—courses of action. Successful resolution is a complex process and requires the care provider to consider many competing alternatives and variables prior to taking action. Situational circumstances may be unpleasant based on involvement of other individuals. Situations that involve promoting advocacy through patient protection, confronting a peer, or reporting situations to authorities can cause feelings of confusion, anxiety, doubt, and even anger for being involved or "placed in such a situation." It is important to be knowledgeable about organizational policies, professional codes, and personal ethical principles and concepts. The nurse must be prepared to think critically in arriving at a resolution to ethical situations.

Framework for Arriving at Ethical Decisions

It is imperative that nurses have the ability to make ethical decisions. Educational programs strive to facilitate this in an effort to produce graduates, and subsequently nurses, who are morally informed, knowledgeable, and accountable. Frameworks for ethical decisions are designed to be used in an effort to enhance the process. They are not designed to be an absolute to decision making, since many factors must be used in coming to an ethical decision. There is no one model or foolproof method that can account for all of these factors in arriving at the "right" decision. An ethical decision involves integration of an individual's personal beliefs and values, use of ethical concepts relative to the nursing profession, and standards or codes of behavior. All of these affect the ultimate outcome and the weight of each may vary considerably based on the situation. In one situation, personal beliefs and values may dominate the equation, whereas in another, the standards or codes of behavior take the front-row seat in the equation. Differences in patient care situations will require different approaches to solving ethical problems. These differences are affected by the values of the decision maker (patient or patient-designated decision maker), the nurse, and other care providers involved in the situation.

Use of the nursing process can effectively be one model for arriving at ethical decisions. This model can be adapted to incorporate ethical components in place of patient care activities and might look like Figure 2. Key questions for each process step can also assist with arriving at an ethical decision (see Table 1).

Table 1. Key Questions for the Nursing Process in Ethical Decision Making

Nursing Process	Key Questions
Assessment	1. What is the client's mental status?
	2. Has the patient been given any medication that would obscure decision-making ability?
	3. Is anyone at risk for physical harm?
	4. What are my values, feelings, and reactions to the client's situation?
Nursing Diagnosis	1. What ethical principles are involved?
	a. Which principle is most important?
	b. Which principle is least important?
	2. What ethical theories are involved?
	a. Which theory is most important?
	b. Which theory is least important?
Planning	1. What do the policies, principles, and codes say about this situation?
	2. Does this situation require consultation with others?
	3. What actions can be taken in this situation?
	4. What actions comply with the most important ethical principle?
	5. Which actions comply with the most important ethical theory?
Implementation	1. Does this plan "feel right: as it is being put into action?
	2. Is this causing more distress for any persons involved as it is being put into action?
Evaluation	1. What were the ethical, legal, emotional, or therapeutic consequences for the patient?
	2. What were the ethical, legal, emotional, or therapeutic consequences for the patient's family and/or significant others?
	3. What were the ethical, legal, emotional, or therapeutic consequences for the health care professional?

Ethical Situation

Scenario: A 36-year-old female is admitted to the hospital for evaluation of a left breast lesion identified on her mammogram. As suspected, it is found to be malignant and she is given the results. She is scheduled for a mastectomy the next afternoon. The patient is visibly distraught and crying. During morning report the day of surgery, the off-going nurse reports that the patient cried most of the previous day and did not sleep during the night. She has also been asking about other options or treatments for "her situation." The night nurse informs you she recommended to the patient that she discuss any issues and questions with her surgeon. She noted that the patient had a list of questions that she worked on throughout the night. When you make morning rounds, the patient asks you about other treatments as well. You reinforce that she needs to speak with her surgeon and that he will be in later in the morning.

When the surgeon comes in to explain the procedure and get the surgical consent form signed by the patient, he is astonished by the volume of questions the patient has and is disturbed that nurses encouraged the patient to speak to him about these questions. He is not prepared to address all of her questions and fails to explain to her satisfaction why surgery is the best option. She decides against the surgery for a few days in order to give herself time to investigate other options. The physician is angry and tells the nurses that this situation is "all their fault." He relays that because

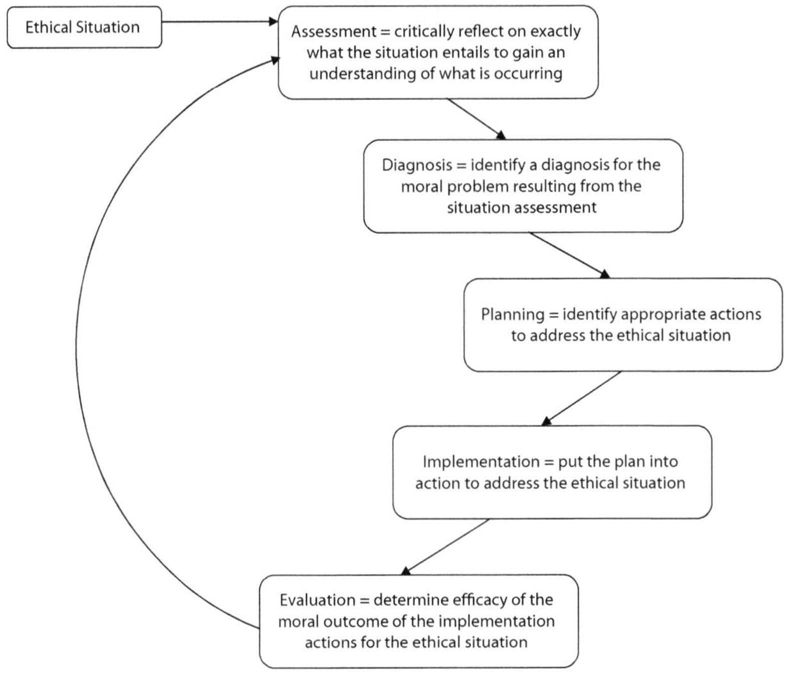

Figure 2. Nursing Process as a Model for Ethical Decisions

of them, the patient may not have the best outcome because she delayed the surgical procedure.

Both nurses meet to discuss this situation in terms of ethical decision making and they use the nursing process grid from Table 1. Their responses are in caps.

Key Questions for the Nursing Process in Ethical Decision Making

Nursing Process	Key Questions
Assessment	1. What is the client's mental status? THE PATIENT IS ALERT AND ORIENTED. 2. Has the patient been given any medication that would obscure decision-making ability? NO. 3. Is anyone at risk for physical harm? NO. 4. What are my values, feelings and reactions to the client's situation? NEED TO ACT AS A PATIENT ADVOCATE AND PROMOTE AN INFORMED DECISION .

Nursing Diagnosis	1. What ethical principles are involved? AUTONOMY, BENEFICENCE, FIDELITY, & VERACITY.
	    a. Which principle is most important? AUTONOMY.
	    b. Which principle is least important? BENEFICENCE.
	2. What ethical theories are involved? DEONTOLOGY, VIRTUE ETHICS, & CONSEQUENTIALISM.
	    a. Which theory is most important? DEONTOLOGY.
	    b. Which theory is least important? CONSEQUENTIALISM.

Planning	1. What do the policies, principles. and codes say about this situation? CODE OF ETHICS FOR NURSES, THE INTERNATIONAL COUNCIL OF NURSES CODE OF ETHICS FOR NURSES.
	2. Does this situation require consultation with others? NO.
	3. What actions can be taken in this situation? PROMOTE AUTONOMY USING THE THEORY OF DEONTOLOGY.
	4. What actions comply with the most important ethical principle? ENCOURAGE THE PATIENT TO SPEAK FURTHER WITH THE SURGEON TO GAIN INFORMATION FOR AN INFORMED DECISION.
	5. Which actions comply with the most important ethical theory? ENGAGE IN ACTIVITIES THAT PROMOTE PATIENT AUTONOMY.
Implementation	1. Does this plan "feel right" as it is being put into action? YES.
	2. Is this causing more distress for any persons involved as it is being put into action? NO.
Evaluation	1. What were the ethical, legal, emotional, or therapeutic consequences for the patient? RIGHT TO INFORMED CONSENT.
	2. What were the ethical, legal, emotional, or therapeutic consequences for the patient's family and/or significant others? INCREASED PSYCHOLOGICAL AND FINANCIAL DISTRESS WHICH COULD LEAD TO FAMILY DYSFUNCTION.
	3. What were the ethical, legal, emotional, or therapeutic consequences for the health care professional? PSYCHOLOGICAL STRESS OF NOT ACTING IN THE BEST INTEREST OF THE PATIENT.

Collaborative completion of this tool served to validate for each nurse that they did the right thing for the patient. If you look at this situation, you may identify different principles and theories. As a result, you may use this tool a bit differently. This is because part of the equation in ethical problem solving is based on the nurse's personal decisions. Neither yours nor the nurses in this scenario are wrong—the decisions are just different.

Summary

It is important to consider ethical principles and theories in arriving at ethical decisions. Managing ethics requires strategic combinations and integration of these principles and theories with understanding in order to arrive at a balance. It involves an integration of knowledge and life skills. Fulghum (1990) said it best:

Live a balanced life—learn some and think some and draw and paint and sing and dance and play and work every day some … When you go out into the world, watch out for traffic, hold hands, and stick together… Everything you need to know is in there somewhere. (pp. 6–7).

From Fulghum, R. (1990). *All I Really Need to Know I Learned in Kindergarten.* Villard Books: New York.

Making ethical decisions is an inevitable part of nursing. These decisions will be independent and interdependent. Patients and families are an integral part of the decision-making process. Nurses must gain theoretical knowledge and work to develop the necessary skills to form a foundation for engaging in the practice of right actions regarding ethics and its consequences on patients, families, and self.

References

Aristotle (1980). *The Nicomachean Ethics* (tr. D. Ross, rev. J. L. Ackrill & J. O. Urmson). Oxford: Oxford University Press.

Banks, S. (2006). *Ethics and Values in Social Work*, 3rd ed. Basingstoke: Palgrave-Macmillan.

Begley, A. M. (2006). Facilitating the development of moral insight in practice: teaching ethics and teaching virtue. *Nursing Philosophy*, 7(4), 257–265. doi:10.1111/j.1466–769X.2006.00284.x.

Bulger, J. W. (2009). An approach toward applying principlism. *Ethics & Medicine: An International Journal of Bioethics*, 25(2), 121–125.

Carr, D. (1988). The cardinal virtues and Plato's moral philosophy. *Philosophical Quarterly*, 38(151), 186—200.

Catalano, J. (2008). Chapter 14: Professional ethics. In *Advancing Your Career: Concepts of Professional Nursing* (pp. 250–267). Philadelphia: F. A. Davis Company.

Chally, P. (1998). Ethics in the Trenches: Decision making in practice. *American Journal of Nursing*, 98(6), 17.

Clouser, K. D., & Gert, B. (1990). A critique of principlism. *J Med & Philosophy*, 15:219–236.

Entwistle, V., Carter, S., Cribb, A., & McCaffery, K. (2010). Supporting patient autonomy: The importance of clinician-patient relationships. *Journal of General Internal Medicine*, 25(7), 741–745.

Fulghum, R. (1990). *All I Really Need to Know I Learned in Kindergarten*. New York: Villard Books.

Ganzini, L., Goy, E. R., Miller, L. L., Harvath, T. A., Jackson, A., & Delorit, M. A. (2003). Nurses" experiences with hospice patients who refuse food and fluids to hasten death. *N Engl J Med*, 349:359–365.

Kennedy, W. (2004). Beneficence and autonomy in nursing: a moral dilemma. *British Journal of Perioperative Nursing*, 14(11), 500–506.

Pagan, N. (2008). Configuring the Moral Self: Aristotle and Dewey. *Foundations of Science*, 13(3/4), 239–250. doi:10.1007/s10699-008-9137-8.

Pollack, J. (2004). *Ethics in Crime and Justice*. Belmont, CA: Thomson/Wadsworth.

Urmson, J. O. (1998) *Aristotle's Ethics*. Oxford: Blackwell.

Vardy, P., & Grosch, P. (1999). *The Puzzle of Ethics*. London: HarperCollins.

Verkerk, M. (1999). A care perspective on coercion and autonomy. *Bioethic*, 13(3/4):358–368.

Williams, D. (2009). Forensic nursing and utilitarianism: The quest for being right. *Journal of Forensic Nursing*, 5(1), 49–50. doi:10.1111/j.1939-3938.2009.01031.x.

Chapter 8: Legal Aspects of Nursing

Nurses are faced with decisions that are affected by legal and ethical issues in their lifetime. Both of these areas of nursing are important for the nurse to know and understand. As health care evolves and society changes in both its health care dilemmas and pattern of health issues, these areas are constantly changing. Technological innovations only add to the complexity of decisions the nurse will make regarding care and outcome or quality of life. This chapter highlights both of these important and complex issues that will be faced by nurses on an ever increasing basis as time moves health care to a more complex interdisciplinary method of care delivery and management.

Legal Aspects of Nursing

Laws in this country originate from the U.S. Constitution, which was adopted in 1787 and is the framework for government organization. This document has as its purpose to: (a) establish justice; (b) provide for the common defense; (c) promote the general welfare; and (d) secure liberty. Laws are rules of conduct that are developed from these purposes and provide for mechanisms to promote conformity to these stated purposes. There are three major types of laws in the United States. These are common law, statutory law, and administrative law.

Common law is also known as case law. This type of law is developed by judges from court decisions. In this type of law, judges use their knowledge of how similar cases have been handled in the past to make legal decisions for current and future cases. The course is bound to maintain the precedent of prior decisions when resolving similar disputes. This allows for similar cases to be decided using consistent principles or rules so that they will have similar results. This type of law is widespread and used in many other countries outside of the United States.

Statutory law is also known as statute law. This type of law is written and formally set down by the legislature on a state or federal level. These develop general propositions of law that courts apply to specific situations when making decisions. A statute may forbid a certain act, direct a certain act, make a declaration, or identify specific government mechanisms to aid society at large. These laws or statutes may be changed or repealed by lawmakers or overturned by a court. Statutes may be time limited and may automatically terminate or be required to be reapproved for continuation.

Administrative law is the group of laws that govern activities of administrative state and federal government agencies. This law delegates authority to specific agencies for the purpose of creating laws that meet statute intent. Actions of these government agencies include rulemaking or the enforcement of a regulatory agenda. These laws may be state or federal. They can address police issues, international trade, immigration, or manufacturing, for example. Administrative laws increase when necessary to address societal, political, or economic issues that evolve over time.

Violation of Laws

There are two general violations that can occur when referring to the law. These include violations of civil law or criminal law.

Civil law deals with the resolution of noncriminal disputes, such as disagreements over property ownership, contractual components, and personal and property damage. Divorce and child custody are also under this type of law. Civil law serves to resolve these types of situations. These disputes may occur between individuals, organizations, specific parties of people or a combination of any of these. There is usually a plaintiff, which is the person or persons complaining about the dispute, or the defendant, which is the person or persons defending themselves against identified accusations. These situations may be resolved without the aid of legal representation in a court of law. Resolution may occur based on state or federal statutes. In other situations, civil law may be based on a court ruling. If no statute exists, the decision in a civil law case may create new laws.

Criminal law is also called penal law as this body of law relates to crime. This law relates to conduct that is prohibited or unlawful because it may cause harm or endanger public safety and welfare. This law also identifies punishment that may be imposed if individuals breach these laws as well. These punishments or sanctions are imposed based on the severity of the violation and can include imprisonment for a designated period of time to loss of one's life for severe crimes against humanity. Elements of criminal law may include punishment of the individuals and a requirement for that person to give back to those who have been harmed (restitution). Some criminal law can extend to include rehabilitation and allow the individual to gain an education and receive psychological help in order to encourage civil obedience upon being released from the prison system (parole).

The Nurse and the Law

The nursing profession holds individuals working within its borders to standards that promote trust by society. These include requirements to practice within the guidelines of the State Nurse Practice Act and civil law. The ever expanding role of the nurse and increasing demands leave the patients open to health care outcomes that may not be desired by patient or provider. It is important for the nurse to be knowledgeable about terms such as malpractice, assault and battery, delegation, informed consent, and patient confidentiality. Even though the chances of a nurse being involved in legal proceedings are small, by exercising one's right to know, the first step is taken toward prevention of poor patient outcomes and subsequent nurse legal issues.

Good Samaritan Act

A good Samaritan is an individual who voluntarily renders aid in an emergency to an injured individual. Even when responding to this type of situation, the nurse is responsible for administering reasonably safe care. In most states, no individual is required to perform first aid unless it is part of a job description. Some states consider it an act of negligence if no assistance is rendered (e.g., calling 911). Some states offer immunity to good Samaritans, which includes protection for errors during the administration of prudent care. This statute does not protect acts that are willful and reckless in the administration of assistance. The good Samaritan law does not apply to individuals performing first aid as part of their duty or job position (e.g., nurse performing first aid in a hospital or clinic). To come under the good Samaritan act, assistance must be given at the scene of the accident or incident and the volunteer must be administering aid without anticipated reward or compensation. An example of a good Samaritan statute that applies to nurses is below.

> When any doctor of medicine or dentistry, nurse, member of any organized rescue squad, member of any police or fire department, member of any organized volunteer fire department, emergency medical technician, intern or resident practicing in a hospital with training programs approved by the American Medical Association, state trooper, medical aidman functioning as a part of the military assistance to safety and traffic program, chiropractor, or public education employee gratuitously and in good faith, renders first aid or emergency care at the scene of an accident, casualty, or disaster to a person injured therein, he or she shall not be liable for any civil damages as a result of his or her acts or omissions in rendering first aid or emergency care, nor shall he or she be liable for any civil damages as a result of any act or failure to act to provide or arrange for further medical treatment or care for the injured person.

From U.S. Legal. (2011). Good Samaritans law and legal definition. Retrieved from http://definitions.uslegal.com/g/good-samaritans/.

Malpractice

Nursing malpractice can occur when a nurse fails to properly treat a patient regardless of setting. This covers actions that are acceptable when compared to other professionals as well. Nursing malpractice is possibly the number one fear of many practicing nurses. Malpractice can cover failure to observe vital signs, failure to monitor or report changes in a patient's condition, errors in patient treatment or care, medication errors that result in patient harm, or any number of care provision activities that are the responsibility of the nurse.

There are two terms that are important for nurses to understand when it comes to malpractice. These include torts, which can be intentional and unintentional, and negligence (see Figure 1).

A tort is a harm done to someone else. In order for a tort to exist, physical, psychological, or economic harm must be the result. These civil wrongs may be intentional or unintentional. Intentional torts are willful acts. These can range from assault and battery to libel (see List 1. Intentional Torts).

List 1. Intentional Torts

- Assault—may be verbal or an offensive contact, e.g., threaten to give an injection without patient consent.
- Battery—any form of intentional touching without patient consent, e.g., actually giving the threatened injection.
- Invasion of Privacy—any form of intrusion (physical or electronic) or dissemination of private information.
- Intrusion on Seclusion—exposure to unwarranted exposure.
- Appropriation of Name—unauthorized use of an individual's name for some benefit.
- Publication of Private or Embarrassing Facts—making public facts that place a person in a shameful situation.
- Publicly Placing One in a False Light—dissemination of facts which place a person in an erroneous perspective.
- Defamation of Character—publication of false statements that result in damage to a person's reputation.
- Malice—publication by a person who knows the information is false but they publish it anyway.
- Slander—harmful statement made in oral form.
- Libel—harmful statement made in written form.

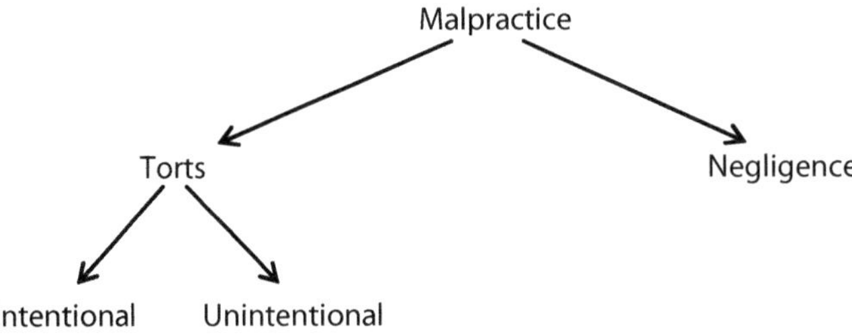

Figure 1. Connection of Legal Terminology

Negligence is failure to exercise the care a reasonable and prudent person would in like circumstances. An example would include a medication error, where the patient was not given their medication at the correct time and a seizure resulted due to absence of this medication dose. A reasonable nurse would check for medication administration times and administer medications as ordered for the patient. Malpractice is a type of professional negligence. There are two prerequisite actions that must be in place before a patient can claim a malpractice action. These include (a) specialized action and skills of the nurse; and (b) through the performance of these specialized actions and skills the patient was harmed. These elements do not just pertain to nurses but to any professional. In addition, for malpractice to be proven, the following four elements must exist: duty (the professional nurse has assumed responsibility for the patient's care); breach of duty (the professional nurse failed to meet the standard of care); proximal cause (failure of the professional nurse to meet the standard of care was the cause of patient harm); and harm (harm or injury is provable).

Nurses with specialized training and extensive experience are held to a higher standard of patient care. This care would be correlated to what a reasonable and prudent nurse with the same training and experience would have done in similar circumstances. Using this standard, a critical care nurse would be expected to recognize potential as well as actual problems and assume responsibility for care. A nurse would be liable in tort if patient harm resulted from an inability to use their knowledge, skill, care, and diligence in nursing care delivery.

As nursing responsibility has increased in complexity, sophistication, and specialization, the role of the nurse to be legally accountable for their actions has also expanded, and so have the expectations of society. Nurses are being held responsible and accountable for actions that promote safe patient care.

Delegation

Delegation is defined as "the act of empowering to act for another." This relates to one person acting for another in the nursing profession. Registered nurses delegate as part of their responsibilities since they are licensed. As part of the scope of practice, they are endowed with this ability in order to accomplish designated care activities. Licensed and vocational nurses are not given delegation authority.

Nurses make delegation decisions every day as part of their care responsibilities. These decisions must be based on the fundamental principle that the outcome will be the protection of public health, safety, and welfare. Effective delegation provides public protection and increases productivity of the nursing care area. It allows for efficiency and continuity of care activities by blending a team of individuals to accomplish specific goals within a designated time frame.

It is imperative that a nurse understand delegation. Even though activities are delegated, the ultimate responsibility rest with the nurse delegating the activity unless the individual to perform the act is also a licensed professional. It is imperative to identify if the person being delegated the responsibility is capable and educated in such a manner to carry out this activity.

The American Nurses Association (ANA), 2001, Section 4.4, gives clear information regarding delegation of nursing activities. See Text 1.

The nurse has significant responsibility as a supervisor of delegated activities. The professional nurse retains legal liability for the actions of the unlicensed individual performing the activity. As the nurse, it is important to know the job descriptions of the individuals being supervised. These will assist in identifying the abilities and approved activities that may be delegated to individuals in specific categories (e.g., licensed practical nurses, certified nursing assistants, etc.). Inappropriate delegation may be grounds for disciplinary action by a state Board of Nursing. As a result, nurses are required to refuse to perform tasks that are not within their scope of practice—regardless of the requesting individual or organization. This is not only a legal issue but it underlies ethics as well. In choosing to delegate, the nurse should consider using

4.4 Delegation of nursing activities—Since the nurse is accountable for the quality of nursing care given to patients, nurses are accountable for the assignment of nursing responsibilities to other nurses and the delegation of nursing care activities to other health care workers. While delegation and assignment are used here in a generic moral sense, it is understood that individual states may have a particular legal definition of these terms.

The nurse must make reasonable efforts to assess individual competence when assigning selected components of nursing care to other health care workers. This assessment involves evaluating the knowledge, skills, and experience of the individual to whom the care is assigned, the complexity of the assigned tasks, and the health status of the patient. The nurse is also responsible for monitoring te activities of the se individuals and evaluating the quality of the care provided. Nurses may not delegate the responsibilities such as assessment and evaluation; they may delegate tasks. The nurse must not knowingly assign or delegate to any member of the nursing team a task for which that person is not prepared or qualified. Employer policies or directives do not relieve the nurse of responsibility for making judgments about the delegation and assignment of nursing care tasks.

Nurses functioning in management or administrative roles have a particular responsibility to provide an environment that supports and facilitates appropriate assignment and delegation. This includes providing appropriate orientation to staff, assisting less experienced nurses in developing necessary skills and competencies, and establishing policies and procedures that protect both the patient and nurse from the inappropriate assignment or delegation of nursing responsibilities, activities or tasks.

Nurses functioning in educator or preceptor roles may have less direct relationships with patients. However, through assignment of nursing care activities to learners they share responsibility and accountability for the care provided. It is imperative that the knowledge and skills of the learner be sufficient to provide the assigned nursing care and that appropriate supervision be provided to protect both the patient and the learner.

From Code of Ethics for Nurses with Interpretative Statements, ANA, 2001, Section 4.4.

Text 1. ANA Delegation

the process of decision making proposed by the National Council of State Boards of Nursing (NCSBN). This process includes

1. Assessing the situation to identify patient needs, consider the circumstances and setting, and assure availability of resources.
2. Plan for the specific task by ensuring that the individual who is delegated the task has the knowledge and skills to perform the task.
3. Assure accountability and validates that the individual delegated the task accepts accountability for their portion of the assignment and understands the task to be performed.
4. Supervise by providing clear directions and validating that performance complies with standards of care and are within organizational policies. Intervene, if necessary, to ensure quality and safety.
5. Evaluate the entire process of delegation which includes the patient, performance of the task, and feedback regarding quality.

This process is circular and allows continuous movement for activities delegated throughout the patient care regimen (see Figure 2).

Because of the increased number of unlicensed individuals in health care organizations, nurses are finding themselves more and more in situations where delegation is a common occurrence and is mandatory in order to accomplish safe, efficient care. The NCSBN also published the Five Rights of Delegation in 1995 in order to address this issue. These rights reinforce the legal and ethical accountability of the nurse when delegating specific nursing care activities. These five rights are as follows:

1. Right task—verify that the care task is one appropriate to delegate to the individual.

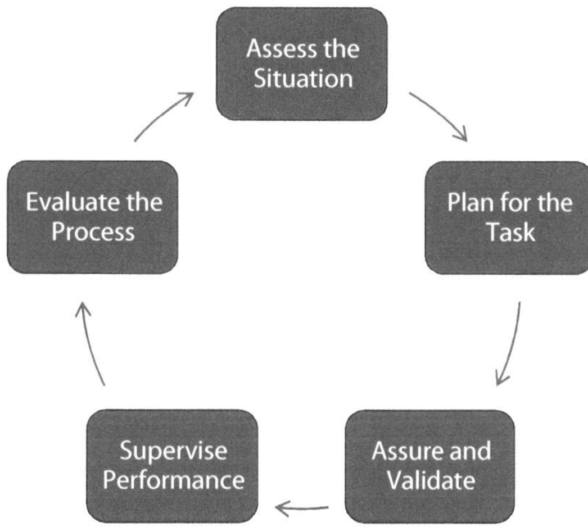

Figure 2. Delegation Decision-Making Process

2. Right circumstances—verify that the patient setting is appropriate, resources are available and all other relevant factors considered in the situation.
3. Right person—verify that the correct persons with appropriate skills and competencies are identified and given the task.
4. Right direction/communication—give clear, concise task description and directions which include task objectives, limits and expectations for completion.
5. Right supervision—appropriately monitor, evaluate and intervene as necessary to accomplish the task in a safe manner. (National Council of State Boards of Nursing, 1995).

Nurses may identify specific task within the nursing process, but accountability for the process itself is strictly held to the registered nurse. It is important for the nurse to know what tasks can be delegated within their realm of responsibility based on their specific state nurse practice act. When moving from delegation to evaluation, knowledge and expertise improve the nurses' chances of effectively using this authority to accomplish safe patient care.

Assault and Battery

Assault and battery is a tort that can result in legal action against a nurse. Assault occurs when there is a threat of bodily harm or an individual is put in fear of being touched without consent. Assault would occur even if there is an attempt to touch another person or a threat to enlist the assistance of others in performing an action against the patient's will. Battery occurs if there is actual physical impact on a person or when a person is actually touched without their permission. If a nurse pushes or slaps a patient this would be considered battery. Forcing a person to eat or take a medication is also a form of battery. As a nurse, in order to avoid potential assault and/or battery it is important to:

1. Inform the patient about care activities prior to initiating them.
2. Verify that the patient understands what the care activity entails.
3. Take time to allow the patient to ask any questions about the activity and consent or refuse the care activity.
4. Make sure the patient fully understands what refusal means regarding the activity.
5. Report refusal to the appropriate person (e.g., charge nurse, supervisor, physician) and chart all facts related to patient refusal.
6. Never impose an activity for a patient against their wishes or desires.

Informed Consent

Many nurses participate in the informed consent process. Informed consent can be written, verbal or implied. In this process, patients have an opportunity to give permission for care activities. Regardless of the type of consent, informed consent must be (a) voluntarily given; (b) given by a competent individual; and (c) received after giving the patient enough information to allow an informed decision regarding the health care activity. Most often consent is in written form for invasive procedure validation in a format that can be maintained in a permanent record. These consents are required for situations such as surgery or invasive radiology. Prior to surgical intervention, it is the responsibility of the surgeon who is performing the surgical procedure to provide information and answer patient questions regarding the specific surgical intervention. It is the responsibility of the physician ordering the invasive procedure to explain the procedure to the patient and answer all questions. Following explanation, it is the responsibility of the nurse to witness the patient's signature and act as patient advocate to verify that the patient understands the intended surgical (any procedure requiring sedation or anesthesia) or procedural (insertion of a chest tube, biopsy, paracentesis, lumbar puncture, radiological procedures requiring contrast or dye) intervention. Verbal and implied consent is routinely sought by the nurse when performing bedside procedures such as vital signs and inserting intravenous catheters. In the procedure explanation the patient has an opportunity to ask questions and understand the need for any procedure. Consent for routine care activities is also included in the provisions of the typical general consent for treatment signed by patients on admission to a health care institution.

The four elements of informed consent include capacity, competency, control, and disclosure. Typically, capacity requires that the person be considered an adult unless they have verification that they are an emancipated minor. Competency involves the ability to comprehend and process treatment options. This means that the person has not received medications or is under the influence of alcohol or a street drug that would alter their ability to be alert and oriented. The patient must be able to assess risks and benefits of the treatment option or intervention they are signing for and note its effect on their overall quality of life. For individuals who are cognitively impaired, mentally ill, or neurologically incapacitated and have a court-appointed guardian or person with power of attorney, then they are approached for consent. Although family members may be at the bedside, they have no legal right to give or withhold consent for treatment for a competent patient. Control is the ability to actually give consent freely and without coercion. Coercion should not be perceived from any health care individual, family member, friend, or acquaintance. Disclosure means that the health care provider must give the patient sufficient information to allow them to make an informed decision. There is no court ruling that precisely states what information the patient should receive, but it must include information related to the nature, purpose, alternatives, and risks for the procedure or intervention. Explanations must be in the language understandable by the patient and the provider must address any patient deficits (vision or hearing).

Informed consent (see Table 1, Procedure for Obtaining Informed Consent) is intended to protect the patient's right to autonomy and self-determination as well as provide validation to the care provider that the patient has given consent for treatment. Decisions cannot be made by anyone other than the patient without verification that another person has legal responsibility and authority to make such a decision.

Table 1. Procedure for Obtaining Informed Consent

Responsible Individual	Task
Nurse	Obtain consent form and have form procedural information completed prior to taking to bedside.
Nurse, with or following physician explanation visit	Go to patient bedside with completed form.
Physician	Explain procedure to patient and others identified by patient to be in attendance. Respond to questions patient may have about procedure
Nurse	Verify that all questions have been answered to the patient's satisfaction. Inform the physician if the patient has new concerns or objections prior to signing the consent form.
Nurse	Sign form as witness to the patient's signature validating authenticity, capacity, and voluntariness.
Nurse	Verify that the form has been placed in the patient's permanent record. Document that the form has been completed and all issues addressed in nurse's notes.

Abandonment

Abandonment means failing to provide adequate patient care until the care of a specific patient is assumed by an approved licensed health care provider. In order for abandonment to occur, there must generally be two components:

1. The nurse has accepted and assumed responsibility for care of the patient (e.g., patient assignment given and accepted).
2. The nurse-patient relationship has been severed without reasonable cause or notice to appropriate persons and arrangements made for care continuation.

These two components validate that the nurse has assumed responsibility for patient care and demonstrate that the care relationship has been severed by the nurse without reasonable notice. There are times when nurses are requested to extend their work hours beyond the regularly scheduled hours. These overtime hours can be consecutive upon completion of an already scheduled shift or in addition to days scheduled. The nurse is expected to exercise critical judgment regarding their ability to accept these hours. They must be able to offer safe care without evidence of sleep deprivation or excessive fatigue. Refusal to accept additional hours or shifts by the nurse is not considered abandonment. Actions that constitute abandonment may vary from state to state but all include patient safety as a critical factor in determining the nurse's responsibility in a specific situation. Some examples of abandonment may include (a) leaving the place of employment during an assigned patient care shift without proper notification and approval; (b) leaving an emergency patient situation, where the nurse's absence constitutes a danger to the patient; (c) not addressing an acute patient situation where the patient is in distress; (d) sleeping while on duty without approval; (e) insufficient patient observation contacts; (f) leaving an organization without giving proper report to the oncoming nurse or approved provider; and (g) failure to report to a facility or care area (e.g., private duty, home care) where the nurse is the sole provider of care without notification.

Confidentiality requires that the nurse safeguard any patient information obtained during care provision and is a fundamental concept in a trusting nurse-patient relationship. Confidential patient information identifies private individual identifiable health and personal information that is often collected in the course of patient historical data retrieval. This could include information related to diagnosis and treatment of past, present, or future physical or mental health situations. This includes identifiable information where there is a reasonable basis to believe that this information can be used to identify an individual.

The American Nurses Association's (ANA) Code of Ethics for Nurses, Provision 3.2, recognizes that nurses have a duty to maintain confidentiality of patient information. "… The standard of nursing practice and the nurse's responsibility to provide quality care require that relevant data be shared with those members of the health care team who have a need to know. Only information pertinent to a patient's treatment and welfare is disclosed, and only to those directly involved with the patient's care. Duties of confidentiality, however, are not absolute and may need to be modified in order to protect the patient, other innocent parties, and in circumstances of mandatory disclosure for public health reasons." (American Nurses Association, 2001) This does not exclude discussion of information with another care provider who has a need to know. It is important to collaborate and share patient information in order to ensure safe, quality nursing care. However, this would not include a nurse or other caregiver who was not involved in the care of the person. Nurses should also only disclose patient information to family members with patient permission.

Patients have a basic expectation that any information they disclose is held in confidence. It is the responsibility and duty of the nurse to respect this expectation. There are state and federal statutes that address the principle of confidentiality. These statutes address privileged communication with individuals such as attorneys and priests. Nurses are not included under privileged communication. If a situation is brought forward in a court of law, the nurse may be required to disclose patient information given to them without patient consent. Nurses should be familiar with their state Practice Act and know any limitations that may exist related to confidentiality in this document. Consistent use of and adherence to specific guidelines can promote safe legal practice by the nurse, related to confidentiality.

Nurses, like other health care professionals, have a duty to report specific situations and not hold this information in confidence. This requirement to disclose information or duty to report includes violations against professional codes, standards of care, and statutes. Professional codes such as the ANA Code of Ethics for Nurses with Interpretative Statements and the International Council of Nurses Code of Ethics for Nurses mandate that nurses take appropriate action to safeguard patients in their care against any action of a coworker that may cause patient endangerment. This includes abuse situations (child or elder), peer conduct, such as practicing while impaired (under the influence of any substance that does not allow care to be delivered with skill and reasonable judgment), or diversion of controlled substances (unauthorized removal of a controlled substance from a patient or facility). Duty to report involving statutes regarding patient situations include certain communicable diseases, gunshot wounds, homicide incidents (gunshot wounds, stabbings, etc.), and OSHA violations that affect patient safety. All situations should be reported to the proper authority.

Health Insurance Portability and Accountability Act

The Health Insurance Portability and Accountability Act (HIPAA) of 1996 was enacted by the U.S. Congress and provides federal protection for personal patient information. This act covers all information held by any health care entity (hospital, nursing home, physician's office, etc.) and communicated in any format (oral, electronic, hard copy). In response to the HIPAA mandate, the Department of Health and Human Services (HHS) published a final Privacy Rule in December 2000 with an April 2001 effective date. This document set national standards for protection of three types of individually identifiable health information: health plans (health insurance companies, company health plans, health maintenance organizations [HMOs], government plans [Medicare, Medicaid, military]), health care clearinghouses, and health care providers (doctors, clinics, pharmacies, dentists, nursing homes, chiropractors) who conduct standard health care transactions electronically. The effective date for compliance was April 14, 2003, with a one-year extension for small health plans. By this date, covered entities were required to implement standards to protect and safeguard against misuse of individually identifiable health information. This Privacy Rule is a foundation for federal protection of protected health information. Organizations must be aware of the ramifications for violations because they include civil and criminal penalties.

HIPAA had as part of its 1996 provision an *Administrative Simplification* requirement related to the development of national security standards for electronic protected health information (e-PHI), electronic exchange, and the privacy and security of health information. The final regulation, the *Security Standards for the Protection of Electronic Health Information* (the Security Rule), was published in February 2003. It set national standards for protecting the confidentiality, integrity, and availability of electronic protected health information. The HIPAA Security Rule deals with compliance addressing three types of security safeguards. These include administrative, physical, and technical. Specific standards and specifications are listed in Table 2.

These standards must be adopted and administered by the organization which identifies the best way to address specifications based on their unique health care situation. Implementation costs can include initiation of sophisticated technologies by many organizations. There was also an increase in required validation and verification, including repetitive charting and duplication of patient information entry. HIPAA safeguards and specifications are listed in Table 2.

The Nationwide Privacy and Security Framework for Electronic Exchange of Individually Identifiable Health Information was published on December 15, 2008,

Table 2. HIPAA Security Rule Safeguards and Specifications

Security Safeguard	Definition	Examples of Safeguard
Administrative Safeguards	Policies and procedures designed to clearly demonstrate how compliance is achieved	• Written set of privacy procedures with a privacy officer responsible for development and implementation. • Policies and procedures that address security controls. • Identified individuals within the organization who will have access to electronic protected health information. • Procedure that addresses employee access to include authorization, establishment, modification and termination. • Ongoing employee training to address protected health information. • Third party (out-sourced) verification of compliance to HIPAA standards. • Contingency plan for emergencies and disaster management. • Internal audits to validate compliance and potential security concerns. • Procedures to address security breaches, risks and vulnerabilities to information.
Physical Safeguards	Policies and procedures to address physical access and control	• Policies and procedures to specify proper use and access to workstations and electronic media. • Access controls to limit use to authorized individuals. • Required access controls to include security plans and maintenance records. • Management of workstation access in public areas. • Policies and procedures regarding transfer, removal, disposal and re-use of electronic media. • Third party (out-sourced) or contractor verification of compliance to physical safeguards.
Technical Safeguards	Policies and procedures to address access and transmission of protected health information	• Implementation of policies and procedures that allow only authorized persons to access electronic protected health information. • Use of controls that prevent intrusion from unauthorized individuals. • Authentication to validate system entry. • Documentation to include access records and technology as well as analysis of risk management programs.

Nationwide Privacy and Security Framework for Electronic Exchange of Individually Identifiable Health Information

by the Office of the National Coordinator for Health Information Technology (HIT) of the U.S. Department of Health and Human Services (HHS). This act is part of the American Recovery and Reinvestment Act of 2009, which provides an electronic health record incentive (EHR) adoption incentive. The timeline for this program is from 2011 through 2014. Principles of the framework guide actions of all health care organizations. These principles are designed to provide for privacy and security protections for individual identifiable health information. Principles include:

1. <u>Individual Access</u> should be provided for individuals in a readable form and format. This is important to self-management of health and wellness.

2. <u>Correction</u> should be provided with a time efficient method for resolution of accuracy and integrity disputes. Accurate information is important for the delivery of safe care.

3. <u>Openness and Transparency</u> should be maintained regarding policies, procedures and technologies that directly affect individual health information.

4. <u>Individual Choice</u> should insure individuals a reasonable opportunity to make informed decisions about the collection, use and disclosure of their health information.

5. <u>Collection, Use, and Disclosure Limitation</u> requires that identifiable health information be collected, used and/or disclosed only to the extent necessary for care delivery.

6. <u>Data Quality and Integrity</u> should be maintained in order to ensure that individual identifiable information is complete, accurate and up-to-date.

7. <u>Safeguards</u> should verify administrative, technical and physical protection.

8. <u>Accountability</u> should be assured through appropriate methods of monitoring.

Office of the National Coordinator for Health Information Technology, U.S. Department of Health and Human Services. 2008. *The Nationwide Privacy and Security Framework for Electronic Exchange of Individually Identifiable Health Information.* Washington, DC.

Nurses routinely access individual patient identifiable health information during the delivery of care. It is important to remember to access only information that is needed to assist in patient care delivery based on the need to know. Entry into the system is confidential and should never be shared. Remember to log out of the system to prevent intrusion by unauthorized persons. Violations for breach of organizational policies that address federal guidelines can result in sanctions that include loss of employment.

Nursing Licensure

Licensure is a police power of the state and has evolved over time in the United States and abroad (see Table 3). The legislative branch of the U.S. government determines which groups are to be licensed and the limitations of such a license. Licensure laws may be permissive or mandatory.

In nursing, the permissive license allows nurses to decide if they will obtain a registered nurse credential after successfully completing an educational program. Permissive law does not protect the title of nurse, but it does protect the use of the title "registered nurse." In order for a practitioner to use this title, they must have completed requirements determined by the state in which they practice. But under

Table 3. History of Nursing Licensure

Year	Event
1867	Dr. Henry Wentworth Acland is the first to suggest licensure for nurses in England.
1893	Nursing leaders organize a meeting at the Columbian Exposition in Chicago to discuss issues affecting nursing, including education and licensure.
1896	American Society of Superintendents of Training Schools for Nurses organize and support licensure in the United States.
1901	New Zealand is the first country to require licensure of nurses; in the United States, New York, New Jersey, Illinois, and Virginia organize state nurses' associations with a goal of enacting a nurse practice act for their respective states.
1903	North Carolina becomes the first state in the United States to enact permissive licensure for nurses.
1915	ANA drafts its first model nurse practice act.
1919	First nursing licensure in England.
1923	All 48 states have permissive licensure laws.
1935	New York passes first mandatory licensure law in the United States (effective in 1947 due to WWII).
1946	Ten states include definition of nursing in licensing act.
1947	New York becomes first state to enact mandatory licensure law.
1950	First year the same examination used in all jurisdictions of the United States and its territories (State Board Test Pool Examination).
1965	21 states have definitions of nursing in the licensing act.
1971	Idaho is the first state to recognize expanded practice in the nursing practice act.
1976	California is the first state to require continuing education for nursing relicensure.
1982	Licensure change to process format examination: National Council Licensure Examination for Registered Nurses (NCLEX-RN).
1986	North Dakota is the only state to require a baccalaureate degree for initial RN licensure and an associate degree for licensed practical nurse licensure (effective in 1987).
1994	Computer-adapted testing initiated nationwide for NCLEX-RN.
1998	Mutual Recognition Nurse Licensure Compact (multistate licensure) finalized. Utah is the first state to become part of the compact.
2011	24 states participate in the compact for multistate licensure.

permissive law, anyone can practice nursing as long as they do not use the title. They may instead use such terms as caregiver or sitter. Permissive law allows the public to identify individuals who have met educational and state requirements and serves as a safeguard for identification by the public seeking someone to function as a nurse.

Mandatory law requires licensure by any person who practices as a nurse. No individual can call themselves a registered nurse without completing required education, successfully passing a licensing examination, and completing state requirements. Initial licensure is the same for all states, but requirements for continued licensure is set by each state and may differ with some requiring continuing education hours and others without this requirement. All states and territories require that registered nurses be licensed in order to practice.

<u>Nurse Licensure Compact.</u> The process of nursing licensure began with each state having its own licensing body; after being initially licensed in one state, nurses had to apply to each individual state for work upon relocating. Due to changing economics, nurse work sites have changed, with some nurses living in one neighboring state and working in another state or nurses working in both their state of residence and a neighboring state. Geological changes and other world events resulting in natural

disasters have resulted in nurse mobility to address societal care needs. Alterations have also evolved from changes in care provision with telehealth (electronic health care) using nurses who live in one state and give care to individuals in another. These evolutionary changes necessitated changes in licensure. The National Council of State Boards of Nursing developed a mutual recognition model for nurse licensure. This model allows nurses to work physically and electronically outside their state of residence and identified licensure as long as that state is a member of the compact. A nurse with an active compact state license is not required to apply or pay fees to any state outside the state of residence in order to practice. Licensure in the home state allows the nurse the privilege to practice in another compact state. Compact states include Arizona, Arkansas, Colorado, Delaware, Idaho, Iowa, Kentucky, Maine, Maryland, Mississippi, Missouri, Nebraska, New Hampshire, New Mexico, North Carolina, North Dakota, Rhode Island, South Carolina, South Dakota, Tennessee, Texas, Utah, Virginia, and Wisconsin. In order to have a compact (multistate) license, the nurse must:

- Reside in a Nurse Licensure Compact state and declare this state as their legal place of residence.
- Meet the licensure requirements in their home or residence state.

Nurses working in a compact state must abide by all the laws and comply with the Nurse Practice Act of the state in which they work. Disciplinary actions may result in the revocation of multistate status, with restriction to the home state mandated.

Nurses residing in a non–compact state are not eligible to practice under the compact multistate license. These nurses are issued a single state-of-residence license. In order to practice in another state, the nurse must hold an individual and separate license in each non–compact state where they desire to practice.

Professional Liability Insurance

Nurses are at risk for litigation claims by patients regarding care delivery. Professional liability insurance, also called malpractice insurance, is a way for the nurse to protect themselves against personal payment for these claims that result in judgment. This insurance for nurses is sometimes afforded through their place of employment, but it may only be active while employed at that organization, so any occurrence that is filed after employment may not be covered by the organization. There may also be a limit to the amount of employer coverage, which means that if the nurse is named in a malpractice lawsuit and legal costs or the final judgment exceeds employer coverage, the nurse may be legally bound to pay the difference. Carrying one's own insurance affords employment portability, continued protection, and additional financial resources. Personal professional liability insurance can protect the nurse while at school, work (primary and secondary employment), and during off-duty emergency intervention.

It is important for nurses to practice responsibly. This means that nurses must be knowledgeable about criteria used for care administration and evaluation. Nurses should possess a copy of their nurse practice act for the state in which they practice, the American Nurses Association's (ANA) *Nursing's Social Policy Statement*, which identifies a definition for nursing and the knowledge base for nursing; the ANA's *Nursing: Scope and Standards of Practice*, which defines clinical practice and its safe implementation; and the *ANA's Code of Ethics for Nurses with Interpretative Statements*, which describes the nine ethical provisions that cover all aspects of nursing practice. Information regarding ANA documents can be accessed through the following website: http://www.nursingworld.org. Using the following 12 DOs can promote legally responsible care by the nurse.

1. DO—know the Nurse Practice Act for their state of practice.
2. DO—adhere to *Nursing's Social Policy Statement, Nursing: Scope and Standards of Practice*, and *ANA's Code of Ethics for Nurses.*
3. DO—be sure to obtain patient signatures when necessary for procedures. Make sure the patient
    a. understands information given by the physician. If not, notify the physician as further explanation may be needed.
    b. has had a chance to ask questions and receive answers from the provider.
    c. understands procedure risks and benefits.
    d. is free to sign or not sign to have the procedure performed.
4. DO—accurately document care activities and results in a factual manner (e.g., medication administration for pain with subsequent follow-up evaluation for level of pain).
5. DO—effectively and carefully delegate care activities using the five rights of delegation.
6. DO—properly make changes to errors in charting. Follow organizational policy when noting errors and making corrections.
7. DO—maintain privacy for patient records and information by knowing laws and abiding by policies related to protection of identifiable patient health information.
8. DO—report allegations of abuse to the proper authority. These include any allegations of physical, emotional, sexual, or mental abuse toward any member of a vulnerable population (e.g., children, elderly, individuals with mental deficits, etc.).
9. DO—use evidence-based research validations for care delivery.
10. DO—use positive interpersonal communications with peers and colleagues to promote communications and interactions that allow for safe patient care delivery.
11. DO—delegate appropriately for the level of the care provider (e.g., peer RN, nursing assistant or care technician, etc.) being given the specific task to perform within the organization and based on organizational policies and procedures.
12. DO—carry individual professional liability insurance.

Summary

Nurses are individually responsible and professionally accountable for the nursing care they provide. Knowledge of legal liability is imperative to protecting patient safety, health, and rights. Knowledge of organizational policies and procedures and the state nursing practice act can promote safe patient care, and are methods that can be used by the nurse to administer legally competent care.

References

American Nurses Association: *Code of Ethics for Nurses with Interpretative Statements*, 2001. Washington, DC: American Nurses Publishing.

Chitty, K., & Black, B. (2011). *Professional Nursing: Concepts and Challenges*, 6th ed. Philadelphia: Saunders.

Hansten, R., & Washburn, M. (1992). Delegation: How to deliver care through others. *American Journal of Nursing*. 92(8); 87–88+90

Harman, L. (May 31, 2005). "HIPAA: A Few Years Later." *OJIN: The Online Journal of Issues in Nursing*, vol. 10, no.2, Manuscript 2.

Healthcare Information and Management Systems Society. (2003). *CPRI toolkit: Managing information in healthcare*. Retrieved August 17, 2011, from www.himss.org/content/files/CPRIToolkit/version4/pdf/4.9.1.pdf

National Council of State Boards of Nursing (1993). *Delegation* (website). Retrieved from https://www.ncsbn.org/323.htm#Delegation_Decision-Making_Process

New York State Education Department (2009). Practice Alerts and Guidelines. University of the State of New York. Retrieved from http://www.op.nysed.gov/prof/nurse/nurseabandonment.htm

Office of the National Coordinator for Health Information Technology, U.S. Department of Health and Human Services. 2008. *The Nationwide Privacy and Security Framework for Electronic Exchange of Individually Identifiable Health Information*. Washington, DC.

Office of Health and Human Services. (2000). Guideline for Compliance with the Standard of Conduct at 244 CMR 9.03(26)—Governing a nurse's duty to report to the Board of Registration in Nursing. Retrieved from http://www.mass.gov/?pageID=eohhs2terminal&L=8&L0=Home&L1=Government&L2=Laws%2C+Regulations+and+Policies&L3=Department+of+Public+Health+Regulations+%26+Policies&L4=Regulations+and+Other+Publications+-+M+to+P&L5=Nursing+Licensing&L6=Policies&L7=Standard+of+Conduct&sid=Eeohhs2&b=terminalcontent&f=dph_regs_nursing_conduct_nurse_duty&csid=Eeohhs2

Robins, Kaplan, Miller, & Ciresi, L.L.P (October 17, 2006). Nursing negligence. Retrieved from http://www.rkmc.com/Nursing-Negligence.htm

U.S. Legal. (2011). Good Samaritans law and legal definition. Retrieved from http://definitions.uslegal.com/g/good-samaritans/.

Chapter 9: Politics and Nursing

Membership in a profession gives one rights and privileges. It also gives them responsibilities that inherently accompany these rights. The focus of nursing is patient centered, but in order to deliver the best care possible it is important for nurses to advocate, educate, and serve as models for the public at large. Often nurses focus on tasks only. Nurses fail to put time and effort into visualizing future directions. Targeting efforts in this one direction does not promote all components of the profession that are required in order for nursing to have the impact it should in societal management. It is important for nursing to promote leadership among its members in order to promote professional credibility and political impact.

Politics and Policy

Politics

Politics can be defined as "the process by which a community's decisions are made, rules for group behavior are established, competition for positions of leadership is regulated, and the disruptive effects of disputes are minimized." (http://www.hyperdictionary.com/dictionary/politics).

This political approach is presented as a system of activity and is concerned with understanding the authoritative allocation of public values and decisions about societal resources (Easton, 1965). A graphic descriptive systems analysis of political life proposed by Easton is seen in Figure 1.

Easton's (1965) approach represents an approach to politics that proposes that a political system has designated boundaries that are fluid or changing. The steps to this approach are presented below:

- Step 1. Alterations in the environment that surround the political system create demands and supports for action which towards the system through political behavior.
- Step 2. Demands and supports for action cause political system competition, which leads to decisional outputs.

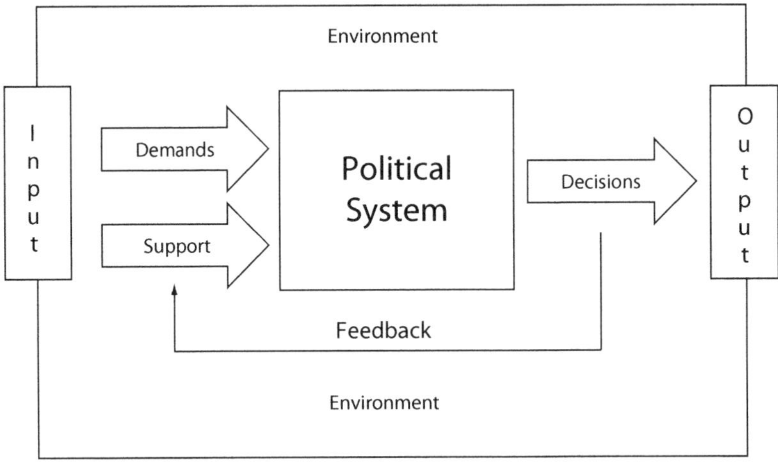

From: Easton, David (1965). *A Systems Analysis of Political Life.* New York: Wiley. Publications. located online in the public domain at: http://en.wikipedia.org/wiki/File:Easton-System_of_political-life.PNG

Figure 1. A Systems Analysis of Political Life

- Step 3. Outputs (e.g., policies) interact with the environment and cause a change.
- Step 4. Environmental output interactions further create group demands or supports for or against the new policy or policy change (feedback).
- This returns the cycle to Step 1 and initiates the cycle again.

This directly relates to how decisions are made regarding resource allocation. Let's look at this system related to health care. No country or community has enough health care resources for 100% of all individuals who reside in that country or community. These resources must be efficiently allocated among individual residents. Demands and supports for action related to health care changes caused political system competition for resources based on specific state, county, and/or congressional district. The health care output in this system occurred in the form of an initiative. One example of an initiative was the Affordable Care Act (March, 2010), passed by Congress and signed into law by the president. This law stated that (a) health insurance companies were to remove out-of-pocket charges for preventive services and give consumers an opportunity to appeal coverage decisions as well as a choice for the selection of a primary care provider; (b) health care costs for consumers and companies must be reduced through implementation of specific actions; and (c) a new competitive insurance marketplace was to be established for individuals and companies. This law was an output that caused a significant change in the U.S. environment. As a result of this change, more group demands were created and supports for and against this law resulted, returning the system back to Step 1.

Incorporated into this system are events and activities that significantly affect whether an initiative gets through the political system. These may be at the national or state level with individuals who are proponents for or against an initiative. They lobby and rally to support their cause and garner support of individuals who have power, influence, or a vote in a certain political arena (e.g., city counselors, state representatives, senators, members of the House of Representatives, etc.) that could affect the outcome of their supported initiative. Individual placement in an elected or appointed position in these situations, give government officials the right to exercise power and influence. Occasionally, this power is not exercised as it should be in the best interest of constituents (see Box 1). This demonstrates the importance for nurses to be involved both directly (running for elected positions) and indirectly (by voting to elect individuals) in the political arena.

Policy

Policy is defined as "a plan or course of action, as of a government, political party, or business, intended to influence and determine decisions, actions, and other matters" (http://www.thefreedictionary.com/policy). These plans reflect values of those involved. Resource allocation is then based on these values. Government policy is a reflection of "a plan or course of action" to resolve specific issues or problems.

At the federal level, government policies are reflected through: (a) constitutions; (b) the chief executive's agenda; and (c) legislative policies. These can emerge as policies or mandates that are then translated into services that reflect a strategic plan or policy memoranda. The plan or policy can be translated into workable components such as rules and regulations, requests for proposals, contractual agreements, etc. Budgets can reflect service decisions based on these items.

Policies are generated from ideas of elected individuals, citizens, or special interest groups. Decision maker values and beliefs also go into this decision equation. Some take into consideration constituent values and beliefs. Ideas that generate policy can result from constituent influences. These ideas result from life events such as parental loss of a child who committed suicide due to being bullied, personal experiences such as a debilitating personal trauma from being hit by a drunk driver, and high-visibility

---

Box 1. Case: Use of Lawmaker Influence

Examine this case that demonstrates an example of influence and why it is important as a nurse to be involved in what happens in the nursing profession. The Board of Nursing in each state regulates the profession. In one southern U.S. state, this ability is under investigation. This is on the heels of a formal suspension of the licenses of three advanced practice nurses due to accusations of overprescribing narcotics. During this period of suspension, the Board of Nursing's right to exist as a regulatory board was up for reauthorization or renewal by the state legislature. At least two lawmakers (state representatives) used their influence to delay the reauthorization vote. These lawmakers used their position and vote—which equaled power—to influence the Board of Nursing to rescind or reverse the three suspensions which occurred prior to the vote for renewal. Following the board rescinding the suspensions, the two state representatives voted in favor of the reauthorization. These lawmakers openly admitted to the press their involvement in using the threat of legislative action to push the state Board of Nursing into reversing revocation of the three nurses' licenses. Following this incident, the state bureau of investigation explored the possibility of official misconduct by these legislators.

issues like health care. These triggers can cause momentum for change and push these issues to the forefront of social concern.

Policies can evolve from philosophies that stem from personal and political values of individuals along party lines. Personal philosophies can be developed in the early years. They learn from exposure to situations and through their education what might, can, and will work along policy lines. Personal philosophies also encourage individuals to identify with specific political parties and organized constituencies. Politicians work to identify and support the will of those they represent. This influences their policy decisions.

Policies may result in laws, regulations, or guidelines that govern behavior in public or private areas. They can evolve from a single constituent idea. Sometimes these constituents are nurses. This was the case with needlestick legislation. Karen Daley, RN, MPH, helped to pass the *Needlestick Safety and Prevention Act (Public Law 106-430, 106th Congress, H.R. 5178) (H.R. = House of Representatives)* of 2000. This requires that health care facilities provide safe-engineered needles/sharps devices for employees providing direct patient care. In 1998, Daley sustained a needlestick injury despite using all the necessary safety precautions. She was stuck while disposing of a second needle in a sharps container. She found out later that she was infected with both hepatitis C and HIV from this injury. This life-changing event led Daley to work toward preventing other health care workers from experiencing the trauma that she experienced. This demonstrates the importance of putting vision into reality in an effort to make work safer for those in the health care profession.

From Idea to Law

There are numerous steps in moving an idea to a specific law. Initial thoughts are generated and written as an idea for a law or rule comes from an individual or group. The following takes you through this process.

1. The idea becomes a bill introduced in either the House or Senate by a legislator in that body. The bill is sent to the clerk of his house, and it is given a specific reference number and labeled with a sponsor's name (bills may be cosponsored). The bill is then read in its entirety (first reading) and the bill is referred to the proper committee.
2. The committee has the power to determine that the idea is not in the best interest of others or unnecessary, which immediately kills the bill. If the bill is identified as credible, it is debated and amendments made if found to be necessary. Following a favorable vote, the bill is sent back to the floor of the house.
3. The bill is now read in its entirety as sent forward from committee (second reading). Members debate the bill and offer amendments. Steps for discussion differ between the Senate and House of Representatives. In the House of Representatives, the time for debating is limited by cloture rules. There is no such standing rule

in the Senate, and individuals can filibuster (talk a bill to death) to defeat it. If successful in the appropriate house, the bill goes forward.

4. The third reading occurs by name of the bill only. A vote is now taken and if favorable, the bill is sent to the other house of Congress (transmitted from House of Representatives to the Senate or the Senate to the House of Representatives).

5. Both the Senate and House of Representatives must pass a bill in order for it to move forward. The bill may be passed with or without amendments. If the bill is defeated it dies in this house.

6. If successful in moving through the Senate and House of Representatives, the bill is forwarded to the president. The president may sign the bill or retain it for 10 days while Congress is in session, after which time the bill will become law without presidential signature. If Congress adjourns at any time prior to the end of the 10-day waiting period, the bill is automatically killed. This action is called a pocket veto.

7. The bill can still become law even after a presidential veto if the veto is overridden by both houses. At this point the bill becomes a law.

The process, though complex, assures everyone that sufficient time and effort is placed on issues that will become laws for U.S. citizens. This demonstrates why it is important to vote for individuals who represent personal values and beliefs. This is a very significant way for citizens to have sufficient influence in politics and on policies.

Getting Involved

Knowledge of government processes is the first step to involvement. Increasing communication and leadership skills also facilitate involvement by adding to one's scientific knowledge and skill foundation. Involvement can take many forms from an individual who desires to directly affect the political scene by running for a political office to an organizational member who promotes changes in a collective fashion.

Individual Involvement
The Nurse as Citizen

Knowledge of issues, laws, and health policy are a starting place for the individual nurse as citizen. It is important to get involved and stay involved at this level by maintaining momentum to move forward and vote for individuals at every election—from local to national. This is a significant way to influence the political outcome on key issues that affect nurses and the health care of those they serve. Political awareness requires continuous monitoring of political stances by elected officials. This can be done through their individual websites, which identify the politician's involvement on issues that relate to the community or country at large. Online access to political information allows any citizen the ability to review activities of the politician, including their accomplishments and votes cast on issues before their legislative body of membership.

The Nurse as Activist

This step moves the nurse from bedside patient advocate to active involvement in political processes. This is a key way to be visible and vocal about health care issues and those that affect the nursing profession. The ideas and issues from the citizen nurse are captured and moved forward to the politician through this mechanism. This level of activity involves lobbying for these ideas and issues in order to let politicians know whether nurses support or do not support these issues and the rationale for their decision. The activist role works with the politician to effect issue outcomes. This was never more apparent than the support nurses provided for Senate Bill (SB) 840 (Single Payer Bill), which was supported in order to guarantee a single standard quality of care for Californians. Nurses made their stand known through activist activities that promoted involvement in rallies, writing campaigns, and phone call initiatives to the governor of California.

The outcome for this bill was not positive, but the efforts by nurses continue to work on health care equity for all individuals. A new activist initiative is underway to promote the intent of SB 840. It is SB 810, the California Universal Health Care Act. As of 2011, it was still proceeding through the political system. This is just but one of the many illustrations of the activism that occurs in states across the country.

The Nurse as Politician

The policy process of idea generation, action to identify potential solutions, and initiation of solution activities is inherent in solving issues relative to the nursing profession. Nurses as politicians are in a unique place to make a direct impact in this process outcome. There is no doubt that the political arena can be intimidating. But nurses have a skill set that makes them effective in political office. Nurses are educated to problem solve using a process that can be adapted to any situation, they learn astute communication skills in managing all types of patient communications that require different approaches for success, they must multitask on a daily basis to address issues as they prioritize them for intervention, and they think holistically in managing patient situations. Besides, on a foundational level—people trust nurses. Putting in the time and effort can be rewarding and beneficial for nurses and citizens alike.

Collective Involvement

Involvement in a collective fashion can start in a nursing program. Many schools have Student Nurses Associations which are part of the National Student Nurses Association (NSNA), with online information located at http://www.nsna.org. This gives you the opportunity to start in a manner that promotes peer support and assistance in developing leadership skills to influence policies at various levels. The organization mentors professional development and serves as a nursing education and career resource. Following graduation, nurses can join the American Nurses Association (ANA) located online at http://www.nursingworld.org. This organization is a broad-purpose professional organization as it is open to all nurses regardless of area of specialization. The ANA represents all nursing interests and advances the profession of nursing by "fostering high standards of nursing practice, promoting the rights of nurses in the workplace, projecting a positive and realistic view of nursing, and by lobbying the Congress and regulatory agencies on health care issues affecting nurses and the public" (from ANA, http://www.nursingworld.org/FunctionalMenuCategories/AboutANA.aspx).

Often nurses work in a certain area of patient care and identify specifically with that type of nursing personally and professionally. As they advance their education, they select a specialized area and focus their career along that path. As a result many will join specialty organizations that allow involvement with this group. These may be focused in such nursing areas as acute care, emergency, oncology, geriatric, pediatric, neonatal, and many more (see a more complete listing at http://www.nurse.org/orgs.shtml). Individual nurses can belong to a specialty nursing organization and the ANA simultaneously. This allows individuals to promote nursing initiatives for the profession as a whole as well as focused in an area of specialization. As a member of both the broad-purpose ANA organization and a specialty organization, standards of nursing practice can be effected on both levels.

Health care is a global issue, and nurses can connect internationally through the International Council of Nurses (ICN), founded in 1899. The organization has three key programs that are called ICN's Pillars. These are professional practice, regulation, and socioeconomic welfare. This organization is a federation of more than 130 national nurses' associations and represents more than 13 million nurses worldwide. This organization is nurse driven and works to ensure quality nursing care for all individuals, promote comprehensive global health policies, advance nursing knowledge, and promote professional respect and satisfaction of working nurses. Membership in ICN is limited to one organization per nation. The nursing organization that represents U.S. nurses in the ICN is the ANA.

Working through local, national, and international nursing organizations can provide a collective vehicle for change. This level of involvement demonstrates a commitment to the profession and society. It allows for unity in the development of public policy. Members allow associations to accomplish their goals and objectives. It is only through the collective work of the members that nursing can protect, promote, and optimize health care for individuals, families, and populations. Some benefits to belonging to a professional organization are presented in Box 2.

Health Equity

Health equity is a global concern. These inequities have been defined as "differences in health that are not only unnecessary and avoidable but, in addition, are considered unfair and unjust" (Whitehead, 1992, p. 430). Health inequities and health disparities are terms often used interchangeably to identify differences among population groups that are defined by specific characteristics. Not only is there inequity in the distribution of health care from country to country, this inequity exists within countries. The United States is not alone in working to address this concern. In order to ensure that this issue is addressed from multiple directions, it is important for nurses to be present at the discussion table. The basis for this unfairness can be attributed to social inequities in opportunities, resources, and constraints that give individuals unequal chances in life (Frohlich, Ross, & Richmond, 2006). These may be related to access to social networks and connections, education which can be linked to economic resources for dealing with health issues related to prevention and treatment (see Table 1). These inequities may be reflected in public policy.

Health care outcomes are based on four broad categories that include personal attributes (biological and genetic), access to health care, health behaviors, and social determinants for health (social, economic, cultural, and environmental). These categories incorporate areas that can and cannot be changed. It is the areas that can be changed that are the ones that affect overall health care and outcomes for disease interventions, with which nurses can get involved. These areas include access to health care through collaborative work with organizations to promote this concept and working with consumers to improve health behaviors.

The next section will address how the United States is addressing this issue through health care reform. Nurses are prime candidates to work in the area of health care reform due to their background in the sciences and patient management.

Table 1. Fundamental Issues in Understanding Health Equity

Area of emphasis	Specifics related to emphasis area
Justice and rights	• Health equity reflects the principle of social justice or fairness to equitable allocation of resources for persons. • Health equity is based on a human rights perspective that includes the right to health and its prerequisites, the right to participate fully in society, and the right to nondiscrimination. • Health equity includes equitable access to health care and the social determinants of health.
Political involvement	• Health involves an interaction between social, economic, material, cultural, and political structures. • Health equity is shaped by policies, which is foundationally a political process. • Achieving health equity requires a multidimensional collaborative approach between interest areas (health care, political, etc.).

Adapted from Reutter, L., & Kushner, K. (2010). Health equity through action on the social determinants of health: Taking up the challenge in nursing.

Social Policy Statement: Nursing's Link to Society

Social policy statements guide decision making. They serve three main purposes: "(1) to operationalize the public's mandate; (2) to establish the professional's scope of practice; and (3) to formulate a framework for influencing health policy" (Gorenberg, Alderman, & Cruise, 1991, p. 11). It is the responsibility of the nursing profession to provide written clarification of its mission, purpose, goals, responsibility, and accountability to the public. Social policy statements serve as the platform for disseminating this information. Nursing is but one part of a larger health care system that is involved with patient care. The social policy statement serves to delineate what part of this system expressly belongs to nursing. The ANA Social Policy Statement serves to define nursing and address issues related to knowledge, standards, and professional regulations. According to this policy, nurses are a critical part of the health care profession and are highly respected and valued for their knowledge, skill, and care delivery (ANA, 2010).

The ANA further stresses the social contract the profession of nursing has with society. The contract is directed toward the nurses' work with all individuals in society, which includes individuals, families, groups, communities, and populations. Elements of the social contract are:

- Humans manifest an essential unity of mind, body, and spirit.
- Human experience is contextually and culturally defined.
- Health and illness are human experiences. The presence of illness does not preclude health, nor does optimal health preclude illness.
- The relationship between the nurse and patient occurs within the context of the values and belief of the patient and nurse.
- Public policy and the health care delivery system influence the health and well-being of society and professional nursing.

- Individual responsibility and interprofessional involvement are essential (ANA, 2010).

As the collective voice for nurses in the United States, the ANA links nursing to society through a social policy statement that addresses key issues inherent in an evolving society. The social policy statement is foundational to establishing the context of nursing, both within and outside of the profession. It serves as a unifying framework for nurses to influence health policy.

Strategies for Political Action

Effecting a change means getting involved. There are many strategies that can be used to promote participation in political activities.

- Become a registered voter and cast your vote in elections. Investigate the candidates and vote for the one who is reportedly the closest to your values and philosophy for health care management.
- Incorporate political science courses in an educational foundation. This is an excellent way to keep abreast of how political activities are being managed, along with the potential to expand expertise in policy and politics specifically related to an area of interest.
- Strategically use the communication mechanisms to keep current of what issues are of importance in the government. This can be done through print media, news releases on television, or online through news and political websites.
- Get involved in organizational committees that form the foundation for effective patient management and nursing practice. Take the initiative to get started. Work closely with an area of interest in order to maintain momentum for a specific political policy.
- Get involved in nursing organizations that promote the welfare of all nurses. Join organizations that are aligned with you as a professional nurse in addition to an area of specialization if that is your desire. There is power in numbers, and increasing numbers in a broad-purpose organization can increase the political potential of the organization and the profession.

The nurse can also get involved in specific activities in order to promote individual and professional initiatives. Be proactive in politics and not *re*active after an issue has been made into law. Many activities can be accomplished without a significant outlay of effort or time. Specific activities can include those in Box 3.

1. Apply to be a Fellow in the White House Fellowship program. This paid position allows participants to work directly with White House staff and high-ranking government officials to effect change in legislative policy.
2. Attend the Nurse in Washington Internship (NIWI). This is a yearly workshop sponsored by the Nursing Organizations Alliance (http://www.nursing-alliance.org/index.cfm) that teaches nurses about the legislative process and how to influence health care policy.
3. Become a member of the American Nurses Association. The ANA is the largest professional organization in the United States that legislates and supports nurses and nursing practice. You can also get involved with specialty nursing organizations that participate in political activities, such as the Association of Women's Health, Obstetric and Neonatal Nurses, the American Association of Critical Care Nurses, or the Academy of Medical Surgical Nurses, to name a few. These organizations develop policies and work to make changes within the health care system.
4. Research health care and nursing issues that are currently being considered by Congress. Start by visiting the online Thomas Library of Congress, a site for federal legislative information (http://thomas.loc.gov/home/thomas.php). Contact the state representative or senator supporting the bill you are interested in to find out ways to get involved.
5. Contact local political leaders. If you are interested in more local issues, you can contact political leaders in your area to learn about current issues and ways to get involved in activities that will support important health care and nursing legislation. Start by reviewing the state website.
6. Start a letter-writing campaign or petition in your hospital or health care organization. This will help to support legislation that is important to your practice. Letters and petitions can be sent to local, state, and/or federal leaders. These give them input to the support or nonsupport of individuals in their area of responsibility.
7. Research the Internet for organizations that support issues in which you are interested. For example, if you are interested in issues related to HIV/AIDS, you could contact the AIDS Institute to assist in activities that will further important legislation, or if you are more interested in patient advocacy, you can contact the Patient Advocacy Foundation (http://www.patientadvocate.org) to locate resources that will support patients and their families.
8. Write a letter to the editor of a local or national newspaper. Use this forum to "spread the word" about issues important to nurses and patients.
9. Write an article for a nursing journal or magazine. This will help to alert other nurses about important political issues.
10. Call local or national radio talk shows. This is a great way to let the public know about important issues. Strategically and effectively communicate your stance on the issues being discussed on the show.
11. Lobby the manager or administrator of your own health care agency about issues that directly affect patient care and nursing practice in your facility. Sometimes starting right in "your own backyard" is the best way to initiate change.
12. Research issues or policies that are important to your practice. Provide a short in-service to coworkers to educate them about the issues you explored.
13. Educate others. Nurses know that educating others is a great way to effect change. For those who do not have the time to participate in "lengthy" legislative activities, simply find a legislative bill or advocacy organization that interests you and send an e-mail about your findings to coworkers, friends, and family. Ask them to pass the information on to others.

Adapted from BellaOnline: The voice of women. Nursing site. http://www.bellaonline.com/articles/art60390.asp

Summary

Learning is a life-long process that involves active engagement. Nurses are responsible for shaping their practice and effecting policies that are important to promoting the best outcome for patients, families, communities, and populations. Developing professional agendas that incorporate active involvement will move the profession forward and promote nursing control over the profession's destiny. Involvement can give individuals a competitive edge because it keeps them informed and engaged. It will also serve to promote personal success and may initiate lasting networking relationships. It is through these relationships that important issues can be addressed in unison and outcomes focused on delivery of evidence-based care at the local, state, and federal levels.

References

American Nurses Association. (2010). *Nursing's Social Policy Statement: The Essence of the profession.* Silver Spring, MD: Author.

Bagwell, M., & Bush, H. (1998). Six steps to better-quality nursing care through political action. *Journal of Nursing Care Quality,* 12:5–6.

Boswell, C. Cannon, S., Miller, J. (2005). Nurses' political involvement: Responsibility versus privilege. *Journal of Professional Nursing,* 21(1), 5–8.

Conger, C. O., & Johnson, P. (2000). Integrating political involvement and nursing education. *Nurse Educator,* 25:99–103.

Des Jardin, K. E. (2001). Political involvement in nursing—Politics, ethics, and strategic action. *AORN Online,* 74, 613–615, 617–618, 621–626, 628–630.

Frohlich, K. L., Ross, N., & Richmond, C. (2006). Health disparities in Canada today: Some evidence and a theoretical framework. *Health Policy,* 79(2-3): 132–143.

Gorenberg, B., Alderman, M., & Cruise, M. (1991). Social policy statements: Guidelines for decisionmaking. *International Nursing Review,* 38(1), 11–13.

Health Disparities Task Group. 2004. Reducing health disparities—Roles of the health sector: Discussion paper. Federal/Provincial/Territorial Advisory Committee on Population Health and Health Security. http://www.phacaspc.gc.ca/phsp/disparities/pdf06/disparities_discussion_paper_e.pdf

Reutter, L., & Kushner, K. (2010). "Health equity through action on the social determinants of health": Taking up the challenge in nursing. *Nursing Inquiry,* 17(3), 269–280. doi:10.1111/j.1440-1800.2010.00500.x

Schutzenhofer, K., & Cannon, S. (1986). Moving nurses into the political process. *Nurse Educator,* 11:26–28.

Toofany, S. (2005). Nurses and health policy. *Nursing Management–UK,* 12(3), 26–30.

Whitehead, M. (1992). The concepts and principles of equity and health. *Int J Health Serv,* 22(3): 429–445.

Winter, M. K., & Lockhart, J. S. (1997). From motivation to action: Understanding nurses' political involvement. *NLN Nursing & Health Care Perspectives,* 18:244–250.

Chapter 10: Technology and Nursing Practice

By Charles W. Revell, MCP, MCAD, MCSD, MCT

Effective utilization of technology is imperative to patient safety in nursing practice. Technological changes are foundational in order to provide continuous quality care, which is at the forefront of nursing practice in today's health care environment. Despite the numerous technological changes made to the health care environment, nurses continue to play a critical role in the delivery of care. They serve as conduits to safety through which technological changes play out their role in delivery of care.

The American Nurses Association defines nursing informatics as a specialty that "… integrates nursing science, computer science, and information science to manage and communicate data, information, knowledge, and wisdom into nursing practice … facilitates the integration of data, information, knowledge and wisdom to support patients, nurses, and other providers in their decision-making in all roles and settings. This support is accomplished through the use of information structures, information processes, and information technology" (American Nurses Association [ANA] 2007, p. 1).

Technological innovations are transforming the culture of care in many organizations. The use of information technologies is one of the five core competencies required of nurses according to a 2003 Institute of Medicine (IOM) document. This impetus gives the nursing profession a fundamental requirement to educationally prepare individuals to deliver care in the technologically based health care organization of the present and future.

Nursing Informatics

Technology is inherent in patient management from entry into the health care system until discharge. In this realm of health care information technology, a need has evolved for nurses who are not only clinical experts. Technologically savvy individuals have the expertise to develop systems but they are not knowledgeable in the language or patient care aspects for which they are developing these systems. It requires a blend of education and skills that include technology and nursing. Nursing informatics is a form of health informatics that applies information technology to the skills and work of nurses in health care. It integrates nursing science, computer technology and information science to effectively enhance the quality of nursing practice. This blending promotes improved communication, documentation, and efficiency in health care delivery by nurses.

Technology promotes fingertip access to information needed to develop individualized plans for patient care management. Integration of technology into nursing allows for an appropriate flow of data collected by nurses in the course of patient management.

From Data to Knowledge

In technology, data consists of characters, numbers, and/or facts gathered for analyses. This analysis can occur at the time of data collection or be deferred to a later time when additional data is gathered for comparative analyses. Data that is interpreted is further moved to the category of information as it is now usable for patient management. One blood pressure measurement alone only gives you part of the patient picture. Correlation of this blood pressure data to prior and current readings allows you to put together information for interpretation and use for effective patient management. From this data to information retrieval, a knowledgeable decision can be made regarding the best course of action for patient management (see Figure 1).

Each level increases in complexity and requires greater application of expertise and intellect to follow through to safe patient care practice and efficient care delivery.

Health care settings are knowledge intensive. Nurses need to exponentially grow in order to effectively use this information. Technology supports knowledge acquisition by allowing just-in-time access to evidence-based information. Nurses have access to this information through handheld devices, stationary and mobile computer setups, as well as bedside computer systems, which allow for retrieval of information that promotes decisions made on the most current research-based information.

Nurses function in several roles in moving data to decision. These roles can extend from foundational to expert. These roles include: (a) data gatherer; (b) information user; (c) knowledge user; and (d) knowledge producer. The data gatherer is an individual whose task is to collect data from patients in various situations. This person can either use the information themselves if they are the nurse or move this information to another care provider who has the primary responsibility to function in other roles of technology movement. The nurse preceptee is new to the health care environment and is just learning to critically think and use information gathered or delivered to them by other care providers. As a new nurse, this person is in transition from the educational facility to full-time care provider using the knowledge acquired over prior years of learning. Through the process of orientation and preceptorship, the nurse learns to coordinate care and organize information for effective and safe care

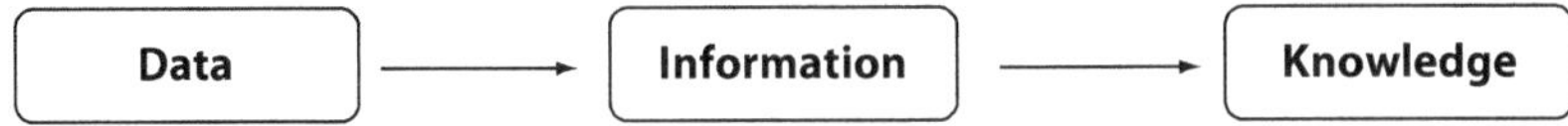

Figure 1: Data to Knowledge Transition

Table 1. Potential Roles and Descriptive Health Care Titles

Role	Health Care Title
Data Gatherer	Nursing Assistant/Novice Nurse—individual who gathers and collects data for delivery to the appropriate care provider, which can include self, in order to promote health care decisions.
Information User	Nurse Preceptee—an individual who is new to the nursing profession and is in the initial stages of using information for health care decisions for patient management.
Knowledge User	Proficient Nurse—an individual who has been in nursing for several years and is capable of quickly moving data through the information stage to knowledge use for decisions that promote safe and efficient care delivery.
Knowledge Producer	Expert Nurse—an individual who has been in nursing and acquired an educational base in a specific area of nursing that allows for correlational analyses and differentiation of data to produce evidence that is research based to promote delivery of care, which is shared with the nursing profession.

delivery. After several years of nursing and after countless hours of experience, the nurse is proficient at delivery of care. This level of expertise allows for development foundational information that can be integrated into a format that promotes individualized care delivery. Information is collectively retrieved and quickly organized into a useable format that allows for on-the-spot retrieval, enhancing decision-making skills. The knowledge producer is a nurse who through his or her years of experience and/or educational background (e.g., certification, higher education, etc.) is an expert in their selected area of nursing emphasis (neurological nursing, hospice nursing, pediatric nursing, etc.). They are capable of expanding nursing knowledge through research and dissemination of the results of their research.

These roles are not mutually exclusive. Individuals may move from role to role based on their care delivery position, movement to another area of nursing (e.g., an experienced home health nurse moving to an acute care surgical setting), and the need to obtain information. For example, the expert nurse may function in all roles when delivering care to a critically ill patient.

In order to make health care decisions, the nurse must be able to access important information when needed. Moving from data to knowledge requires that the nurse have access to critical information at a moment's notice. It is important that the system in place afford nurses the ability to retrieve and manage information. With nursing involvement, this integration of critical information and system usability will be promoted. It is the nurse's responsibility to learn how to effectively access this information for the best possible outcome for patient management.

Electronic Records and Care Delivery

Most health care organizations have computerized systems for some part or all of care documentation. This can range from such services as laboratory and radiological information to total documentation of care by nurses at the bedside or point-of-care delivery. The end result can be a totally paperless system that requires awareness of information flow and management by the nurse.

Electronic patient-based records are also known as electronic medical records, electronic health records, electronic patient records, or computerized patient records. All of these terms refer to a systematic collection of patient-based information. The Health Information Management Systems Society's (HIMSS) defines the Electronic Health Records as "a longitudinal electronic record of patient health information generated by one or more encounters in any care delivery setting. Included in this information are patient demographics, progress notes, problems, medications, vital signs, past medical history, immunizations, laboratory data, and radiology reports. The EHR automates and streamlines the clinician's workflow. The EHR has the ability to generate a complete record of a clinical patient encounter, as well as supporting other care-related activities directly or indirectly via interface—including evidence-based decision support, quality management, and outcomes reporting."

Electronic patient-based information may be static or dynamic. Static records include information placed in a record at a designated time, such as during a wellness physician visit and not updated hourly or daily. These records remain in a database state until acted upon at a specific time. Some examples of these include patient demographic data and prior health historical information. Dynamic records are those that accept constant input of information from seconds to minutes or hours. These are used in care facilities that require continuous input of information. Some examples of these include information entered in acute care settings, such as vital signs, procedures, laboratory data, etc. Regardless of the type of record, it can be shared across different health care settings and give instant access to critical information needed for care decisions by nurses and other care providers.

Each patient encounter results in the capture of data. The electronic health record network integrates data from all participating systems (e.g., administration, nursing, laboratory, radiology, pharmacy, etc.) and organizes it to create the EHR for a specific patient. This information can then be retrieved for coordination of care (see Figure 2).

Future EHRs will incorporate the ability for nurses to retrieve patient data from a multitude of sources inside and outside their organization. It all incorporates supporting security measures that allow for access across organizational, state, and country of origin boundaries. This system will be nationwide and worldwide, integrating

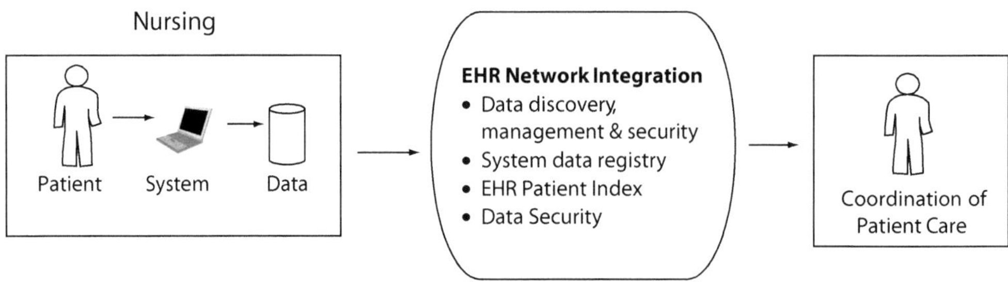

Figure 2. Electronic Health Record (EHR): Nursing Concept Overview Nursing

translational components to allow for enhanced operation across nationalities and cultures.

Information Security

Security in the information technology world is a significant issue. Security must ensure that the Health Insurance Portability and Accountability Act (HIPAA) is addressed in an effort to provide continuity of care without risk to health information for patients. Information for health care crosses many areas within acute and extended care facilities, physician offices, outpatient settings, and others. It is important that security be addressed in an effort to assure access in an effort to improve quality of care, prevent medical errors, reduce paperwork, and expand access for individuals seeking care.

Measures to control threats and vulnerabilities in information systems can be organized into three categories of safeguards. These include administrative, physical, and technical. HIPAA security standards fall in the administrative category. These administrative safeguard actions, policies, and procedures manage the selection, development, implementation, and maintenance of measures that manage patient information (Department of Health and Human Services, 2003). Physical safeguard actions include policies, procedures, and measures that control physical access to information devices that house information such as computers, servers, networks, and buildings where devices that house information are stored. Technical controls include devices associated with security of information. These include passwords, firewalls, and encryptions that assure integrity of patient health information.

Security is imperative in health care in order to protect the rights of individuals regarding their health information. Organizations must ensure that security addresses confidentiality, integrity, and availability of information. A patient data system must be secure in that it does not allow information to undisclosed individuals. Access must be restricted to individuals who have no "right to know." Systems must be password restricted and partitioned in segments that give specific individuals access to designated information. The system must have data integrity. Information must be correct and unalterable by persons without specific access and privileges. This ensures that information is correct as entered and does not allow misrepresentation of information in the system. Availability is the property that data or information is accessible and usable on demand. In health care, it is imperative to be able to access specific information when necessary to ensure continuity of patient care.

Nursing's responsibility for security encompasses user awareness. Nurses gain entry to patient health care information systems through passwords, specific system keys, or other security components. When logging in or accessing the system for input, alteration, or review of patient information, it is imperative to logout or return the system to a user-ready state. This prevents access by unauthorized individuals under another's specific user information. Consistent awareness of the general extent of security measures, practices, and procedures for security of the system is a must. It is the ethical and legal responsibility of all health care professionals to protect patient information from unauthorized access.

Patient Safety

Patient safety is of utmost concern in health care. Keeping the patient safe through the reduction of accidental injury is part of a nurse's responsibility. Errors can be costly in terms of quality of life for patients and families and fiscal recovery from an organization for such errors (e.g., judgment against an organization by a court system or federal/state fines for not adhering to safe practice standards). Patient safety is not only a responsibility of the nurse but has been championed by other organizations in an effort to reduce the number of errors and subsequent negative outcomes. In 2000 the Institute of Medicine (IOM) published a landmark report that heightened public awareness of health care errors. According to this report, as many as 98,000 Americans die in hospitals from medication errors. Many occurrences are due to human error, and in an industry where service from people is a standard, it is important to address these errors. One strategy identified in the IOM publication is the use of technology to address these errors. Technology can be used to promote safe care activities through

1. Use of prompts to identify inconsistencies or alerts in a computerized system (e.g., an alert for a medication that is ordered that is on a patient's allergy list, inappropriate medication dose alert, retrieval of blood pressure or heart rate prior to administration of a specific medication, etc.).
2. Use of constraints or forcing functions, which require that the individual act on a presented situation before being allowed to progress to the next action.
3. A "plan for recovery" system that would allow for reversal of an operation with validation such as deletion or moving information within the system
4. Standardization of actions that would require the use of preset protocols in order to complete an action.

The use of technological innovations can reduce unsafe patient situations and the occurrences of what are called sentinel events in patient care. A sentinel event is one where an unexpected situation occurs, which places a patient at risk for death or actually results in death or serious physical or psychological injury. An example of serious physical injury might include discharge of an infant to the wrong family, medication error that results in death or major permanent loss of function, or a patient fall that results in death or major permanent loss of function. A psychological injury might include a stress-related emotional condition resulting from real or imagined threats such as an event that might cause substantial and lasting psychological damage, such as depression or significant anxiety. These events are termed "sentinel" because they identify an immediate need for investigation and response by the organization. Nurses should be proactive in embracing a technology that promotes patient safety through early identification and alert systems. These systems serve to identify needs that require immediate action.

Informatics Competencies

Competencies have been identified by the ANA (2007) regarding informatics for nurses. These levels are (a) entry level; (b) experienced nurse; (c) informatics nurse; and (d) informatics nurse specialists. They promote a leveling that allows nurses to identify where they are on the knowledge scale of information technology. This knowledge encourages further acquisition in order to understand the intricate skillset required for the use of technology in health care.

Entry Level

Skills include those basic to computer use such as keyboard skills, document management, accessing hardware such as thumb drives and headsets, etc. These skills extend to electronic communication in the form of e-mail skills from message generation, use of appropriate tone for communication, and forwarding information from one individual to another. Word-processing skills are also elementary to communication, as they include the ability to generate, edit, and save information in document format, allowing for later retrieval and use. Web skills are also needed as an entry level skill in order to search and capture information required for evidence-based validation of patient care. This information may also be downloaded and maintained in a format for quick identification and retrieval by the user. These skills are foundational to clinical and administrative processes that nurses use in their daily activities (see Table 2).

Accessing information for patient management is part of the necessary skill of the entry level nurse. Data is important to decisions that are made for implementation of care and in relaying patient information to peers and other health care providers throughout the course of patient management.

Experienced Nurse

The experienced nurse expands on skills of the entry level nurse. In addition to possessing entry level skills, this nurse supports their specific specialty area with quality improvement activities and other activities to promote safe and skilled patient care

Table 2. Processes That Support Nursing Activities

Processes	Activities
Clinical Processes	• Working with computers in various formats for input of patient data: (a) immobile (stationary); and (b) mobile (Computers on Wheels [COWs] or Workstations on Wheels [WOWs). • Retrieval of patient record components (e.g., laboratory tests, electrocardiograms, radiological tests).
Administrative Processes	• Accessing physician orders for implementation. • Patient triage (e.g., movement of patients who are less critical for admissions who have a higher acuity) and bed management for admitted patients.

using technology. This level of informatics nurse uses evidence-based databases to promote high-level nursing care activities for patients. Through the promotion of technology applications, the nurse can improve patient outcomes. The experienced nurse works with the organization's information technology department to promote system improvements. These improvements allow for nurses to deliver quality, safe care to patients in all environments.

Informatics Nurse

The informatics nurse possesses entry level and experienced informatics nurse skills. They also possess all the skills required to be proficient with technology applications used to support all areas of nursing practice. They are engaged in fiscal management for hardware and software integration within the organization. They are skilled in data management, system development, and use of computer applications. Their involvement in data management may include data design or the way data is structured in the organization's system, data storage, which refers to the many ways data can be stored (e.g., hard drives, flash memory, optical media, or temporary Random Access Memory [RAM]) and/or data security that involves management of firewalls or other security encryptions that may exist to maintain data and system integrity.

Informatics Nurse Specialist

The Informatics Nurse Specialist possesses all prior skills and has an in-depth understanding of the various levels of technology. This extends from the user interface to mainframe security technology. This individual conducts research and generates theoretical foundations for informatics nursing. This nurse is pivotal to evidence-based validation of technology-based solutions that improve nursing communication and increase the efficiency of patient care. This individual is often a member of the multidisciplinary team for an organization that promotes integration of computer technology to improve patient care. The Informatics Nurse Specialist often promotes strategic planning and determination of system solutions that support patient care. This individual works to develop standards for technology use in clinical applications while conforming to organizational accreditation standards and regulatory requirements.

Informatics and Nursing Care

Information technology is a cornerstone of patient safety and continuity of care. Clinical decision support systems (CDSSs) are key applications driven by information technology. They are computer software applications that match patient characteristics with a knowledge base to generate specific guidelines for patient management. CDSSs are associated with advancements in evidence-based practice and continuity of care. A CDSS could be used by nurses at the bedside to access critical information that would aid in moment-to-moment decisions that could include historical information and current treatments in graph format, which would demonstrate trends. CDSSs generate information and facilitate the generation of guidelines to support decisions made by the nurse as care provider.

In their 2001 document *Crossing the Quality Chasm: A New Health System for the 21st Century*, the Institute of Medicine identified redesign imperatives for health care in order to provide safe, effective, patient-centered care. These redesign imperatives are:

1. Reengineered care processes.
2. Effective use of information technologies.
3. Knowledge and skills management.
4. Development of effective teams.
5. Coordination of care across patient conditions, services, and sites of care over time.

The second of these is the effective use of information technology. In order for this to occur, nursing must be capable of working within this computerized system to administer care that is dependent on the use of information technology for patient care delivery. Computer technology holds enormous potential but requires an infrastructure that promotes health care delivery by all care providers, patient health, quality measurement and improvement, and clinical research and education. This commitment would require the adoption and effective use of information technology applications in all sectors of health care. Effective implementation of technology in nursing care would require behavioral adaptations regarding patient care management. These adaptations would allow the nursing profession to promote technology use in building a strong base of support for administering high-quality, safe, effective, patient-centered care.

Summary

Technology unfolds over time and allows for improved access to patient information at the point of care and enhances nursing's abilities to benchmark, monitor, and audit quality measures. As technology users, nurses will mature in their use of innovative technologies that promote the delivery of high-quality care. With nursing informatics, the passion for nursing, technology, and innovation leads to improved patient outcomes and higher quality patient-nurse interactions.

Allan, J., & Englebright, J. (2000). "Patient-Centered Documentation: An Effective and Efficient Use of Clinical Information Systems," *Journal of Nursing Administration.* 30(2):90-95, February 2000.

American Nurses Association. (2007). *Scope and Standards of Nursing Informatics Practice.* Silver Spring, MD: Author.

Barton, A. J. (2005). Cultivating informatics competencies in a community of practice. *Nursing Administration Quarterly, 29*(4), 323-328.

Booth, R. G. (2006). Educating the future e-health professional nurse. *International Journal of Nursing Education and Scholarship, 3*(1), 1-10.

Department of Health and Human Services. (2003). Final Security Standard, Title 45 CFR Parts 160, 162, and 164, www.cms.hhs.gov/hipaa/hipaa2/regulations/security/03-3877.pdf.

Hebda, T., & Czar, P. (2009). Handbook of Informatics for Nurses and Healthcare Professionals. 4th ed. New Jersey: Pearson.

Institute of Medicine (IOM). (2000). To err is human: Building a safer health system. Washington, DC: National Academy Press. Retrieved from http://www.nap.edu/openbook.php?record_id=9728&page=R1

Institute of Medicine (2001). Crossing the quality chasm: A new health system for the 21st century. Washington, DC: National Academy Press. Available at http://www.nap.edu/openbook.php?isbn=0309072808

The Joint Commission. (2011). Sentinel event. Retrieved from http://www.jointcommission.org/sentinel_event.aspx

Chapter 11: Nursing Education

The Path to a Nursing Career

I n order to achieve the goal of becoming a nurse, one must select a route and educational delivery that supports their ability to learn information and fit within their overall personal life situation. The educational process of the nurse can take many routes. Even after successfully completing a basic education, the nurse must be licensed in order to administer care. This two-step process—education and licensure—are an introduction to the lifelong process of learning that the nurse undertakes.

Nursing's Educational Pathways

One may enter the nursing profession in one of three ways. These include a diploma program, an associate degree program, or a baccalaureate degree program. All programs offer theoretical and clinical components. These programs are different in their basic educational preparation, which includes length of the program and number and type of courses offered, affecting the cost of each program type. Upon successful completion of a basic education, the new graduate is eligible to take the National Licensing Examination for Registered Nurses (NCLEX-RN) in their state of choice, as all states have the ability to offer the examination. When successful, the graduate can legally use the credential RN and practice as a registered nurse in a health care setting of their choice.

The pre-licensure educational route from student to RN can be achieved by one of three different routes (see Figure 1). It is not uncommon that nurses prepared through all educational routes work side by side. This can be confusing for many individuals receiving health care from a registered nurse, as these nurses may work side by side in the health care delivery system.

The most common route for entering the nursing profession reported since 1996 to 2008 has been the associate degree program (see Figure 2). The number of graduates prepared at the diploma level has steadily declined since 1980. The number of nurses prepared at the baccalaureate degree has increased, although this trend has not matched or surpassed the associate degree route. Some programs have evolved that prepare nurses at higher levels. There are programs that promote completion of education with educational termination at the master's or doctoral level. These

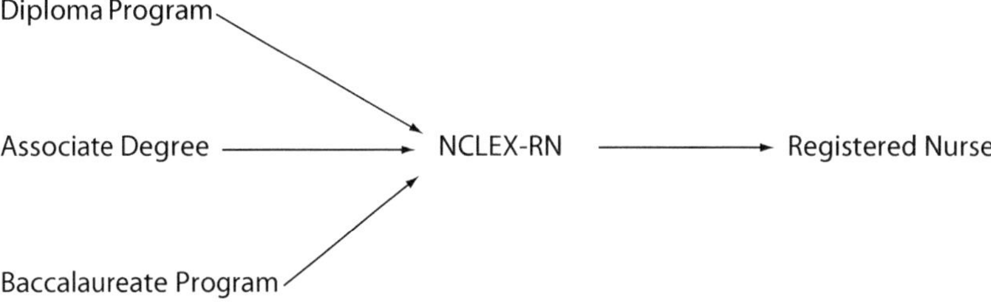

Figure 1. Educational Route for the RN

programs are usually promoted for individuals with some previous educational experience or degree. These individuals have a history of completing a postsecondary educational experience or working in a field outside of nursing. They allow entry at an advanced level into the academic process and upon completion of a designated program of study, the individual can exit the higher educational institution with a master's or doctoral degree in nursing. These programs are still small in number.

Diploma Program

Diploma or hospital-based programs in nursing were the first U.S. programs for nurses. These appeared in the late 1800s and transitioned from the Nightingale School in 1860 in England. These schools spread quickly and grew to approximately 2000 by 1930. Programs used the fundamental hospital as a training laboratory, and this allowed these organizations to reduce labor costs for nursing staff. These programs had some classroom learning activities, but most were delivered in an apprenticeship format. Classroom and clinical activities were often combined in a 24-hour day, with minimal time for rest and relaxation. Courses were offered in areas of nursing currently used, as these correlated to the medical model which was familiar to many hospitals. Obstetrics, pediatrics, and surgery were among courses offered over the three-year study period. This allowed the hospital to have students deliver care throughout the 24-hour period, seven days a week. Nurse graduates were awarded a diploma upon successful completion of the program, since these schools could not grant academic credit for a degree.

Following transition from a hospital-based program to an academic setting, the numbers of diploma programs significantly declined in the mid-1960s. These numbers continued to decline through 2000, with only 62 programs reported. This decline was in part due to the growth of associate and baccalaureate programs, and some diploma programs were actually phased into these programs. Changes in health care financing and fiscal reductions for organizational education also caused the closure of some programs. Program requirements also changed with the transition to academia. State requirements for operating schools of nursing were required to be met in order to prepare students for success on the state licensure examination.

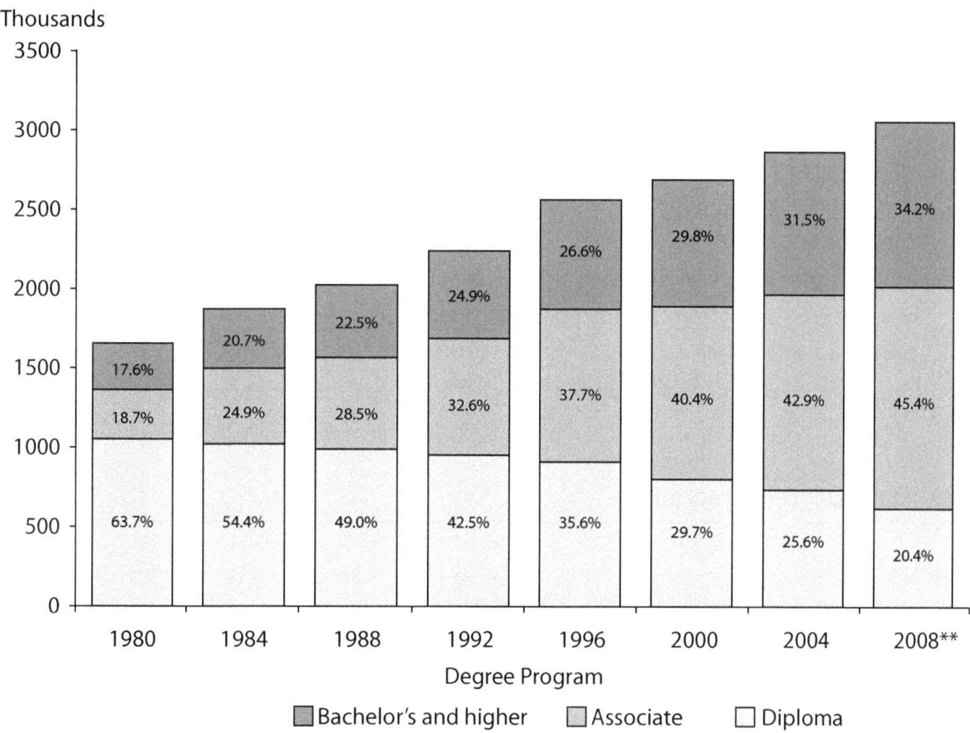

* The counts for all initial degrees may not add to the total registered nurse estimates for each survey due to incomplete information provided by respondents and the effect of rounding. Only those who provided education preparation information are included in the calculations used for this figure.

**For 2008 initial education—13,325 were registered nurses with master's degrees (0.4%) and 954 with doctorate degrees (0.03%).

From the U.S. Department of Health and Human Services Health Resources and Services Administration (2010). *The registered nurse population. Findings from the 2008 national survey of registered nurses.* Retrieved from http://bhpr. hrsa.gov/healthworkforce/rnsurveys/rnsurveyfinal.pdf

Figure 2. Distribution of Registered Nurses according to Initial Education, 1980 to 2008*

Nurses who graduated from diploma programs were at a disadvantage when they desired to continue their nursing education. Hospital-based courses were not offered by an organization that was part of the higher education system. In an effort to expand opportunities for diploma graduates, some programs developed articulation agreements with universities and colleges. Alignment with these programs of higher education promoted transition to associate or baccalaureate degree programs, with some academic credit toward degree completion upon successful completion of the diploma program.

Many diploma programs are now accredited by the National League of Nursing (NLN). As of 2011, there were 59 accredited diploma programs. Accreditation validates that the program meets standards for

1. Mission and administrative capacity—that the mission and core values are congruent with strategic goals and objectives between the educational unit and governing organization.
2. Faculty and staff—faculty and staff provide the necessary leadership and support for the academic unit to attain goals and outcomes.
3. Students—policies, development, and services for students support goals and outcomes.
4. Curriculum—prepares students to achieve identified outcomes.
5. Resources—sufficient fiscal, physical, and learning resources exist to achieve goals and outcomes.
6. Outcomes—evaluation demonstrates achievement of identified competencies.

Associate Degree Programs

Associate degree programs in nursing have seen a steady increase over diploma or baccalaureate degree programs. These numbers increased from just three programs in 1952 to a little more than 1,000 by 2008. The length of time and ability to compete for some nursing positions boosted the desire to attend these programs. Programs are usually two years in length compared to the four years of a baccalaureate program. The AND program offered additional incentives to attend, including part-time study, financial affordability, and access or proximity to the growing number of programs. The educational development of these programs were a direct result of a model for education developed by Dr. Mildred Montag. This model was an attempt to address the nursing shortage following World War II. The Montag Model identified a bedside nurse who was dedicated to performing nursing functions without administrative responsibilities. The functions of this nurse focused on

1. Assisting with planning nursing care activities;
2. Giving supervised general nursing; and
3. Assisting in evaluation of nursing care activities.

The model proposed by Montag has changed over the years, and the curricula of the AD-prepared nurse may now include courses that address leadership and clinical decision making. These courses are outside the original model proposed by Montag and may increase the program of study to more than two years. These programs now graduate nurses that are difficult to differentiate from baccalaureate graduates in function and employment setting. Many work as peers to both diploma and baccalaureate degree graduates. Some even assume charge or head nurse positions in health care organizations.

The associate degree nurse graduate may transition seamlessly into the baccalaureate program of study. As a result of associate degree courses being in academic settings (unlike diploma graduates), some of the courses taken by the associate degree graduate may be recognized in the baccalaureate program of study. Articulation agreements with baccalaureate programs facilitate this transition in some AD programs.

The NLN Council of Associate Degree Programs first proposed to differentiate competencies for the associate degree nurse from those of the baccalaureate degree graduate in 1990. The document was revised in 2000 in order to address changes in an evolving health care system. This document identified eight core competencies which included

1. Professional behaviors;
2. Communication;
3. Assessment;
4. Clinical decision making;
5. Caring interventions;
6. Teaching and learning;
7. Collaboration;
8. Managing care.

These core components emphasize competencies related to diversity in health care, clinical decision making, assessment, patient education, continuity of care (including community aspects), collaboration, and leadership. The ADN graduate is designed to be a generalist upon successful completion of a program of study.

Baccalaureate Degree Programs

The first baccalaureate degree program was established in 1909 at the University of Minnesota. This program resulted from research that promoted a move for nursing education to shift from a hospital-based educational component to colleges and universities. Nursing leaders identified that this educational foundation was needed to promote nursing as a profession. It was felt that a bachelor of science in nursing (BSN) degree would prepare graduate nurses to assume leadership positions.

Since initial program inception, BSN programs have continued to develop at universities, and allow individuals the opportunity to obtain a degree and prepare for nursing licensure simultaneously. Courses in a BSN program of study include liberal arts, science, and nursing. Many programs are structured to allow for electives in these areas. This permits the individual to select courses that work to complete a minor study area if desired. Nursing courses focus on various settings that include public or community health. Extending skills in this area promotes independence while managing patients in the public or community health setting. This area is unique to the baccalaureate degree curriculum.

Nurses may enter BSN programs as extensions of their program of study as the basis of their initial RN licensure. In some programs, RNs receive credit for prior education and/or experience. This may be achieved through validation of prior education on a transcript from an educational institution or by successfully challenging knowledge in an area by examination. Often, programs are flexible to permit part-time education as the nurse continues to work. Some programs offer courses outside of typical on-ground classroom settings, with many offering them in a full or partial (hybrid) computer-based or online format.

In 1965 the American Nurses Association (ANA) published a position paper that addressed educational preparation. This document was foundational in defining nurse graduate knowledge, skills and values. The association's first position paper entitled *Educational Preparation for Nurse Practitioners and Assistants to Nurses* made four major recommendations. These were

1. Education for all who are licensed to practice nursing should take place in institutions of higher education,
2. Minimum preparation for beginning professional practice should be baccalaureate degree education in nursing,
3. Minimum preparation for beginning technical practice for nursing should be associate degree education in nursing, and
4. Education for assistants in the health service occupation should be a short, intensive preservice program in vocational education institutions rather than on-the-job training programs. (ANA, 1965)

The 1965 position document was not widely accepted by those inside or outside of the nursing profession. Many nurses were educated at the diploma level, and there was no recognition of these nurses in the document. The document would require a new manner of thinking and have unique regulatory and licensure implications. This brainstorm of responses spanned the continuum of acceptance to rejection. It segmented nurses into those who could use the terms professional and RN from those who could not. The term "technical" was interpreted to mean a level below the one currently occupied by associate degree nurses. It was also interpreted to mean that these nurses would have limited responsibilities related to patient care. Many organizations devoted much time and energy addressing both ends of the acceptance continuum.

In 1970 a new document entitled *An Abstract for Action* was published by the National Commission for the Study of Nursing and Nursing Education. This document presented the outcome of a study that addressed nursing practices and patterns and the assessment of future needs. Four key recommendations from this study centered on (a) the need for resources to study nursing's practice impact on health care; (b) establishing state master plans to ensure that nursing education is positioned in educations mainstream; (c) the formation of a National Joint Practice Commission and state counterparts; and (d) the adoption of governmental measures to support research in nursing. This document did not defuse all controversy related to nursing's educational foundation. Comments included criticism about the research process, which made results less than credible or perspectives that the study offered no new information for the nursing profession.

In 1979 the ANA placed a timeline on preparation and differentiation of nursing. They proposed that changes to the entry level of nursing practice be the baccalaureate degree by 1985. Nursing should be identified by two levels (professional and technical) by 1980, with competencies identified for each level. Accessibility was also identified as a component to be addressed that would allow for career mobility, with flexibility in approaches to addressing this issue. The 1980s saw these dates come and go with no action by the profession.

Baccalaureate degree programs were challenged by the American Association of Colleges of Nursing with their 1986 document to ensure the abilities of their graduates. The document entitled *Essentials of College and University Education for Professional Practice* discussed nursing's context and its effect on student education and socialization. It identified abilities that baccalaureate degree programs should ensure in their graduates. These included the following:

1. Read, write and speak English clearly and effectively to acquire knowledge, convey and discuss ideas, evaluate information and think critically.
2. Think analytically and reason logically using verifiable information and past experience.
3. Understand a second language at a minimum of an elementary level to widen access to diversity.
4. Understand other cultural traditions to gain perspective on personal values and similarities and differences among individuals and groups.
5. Use mathematical concepts, interpret quantitative data and computers and other information technology to analyze problems.
6. Use concepts from the behavioral and biological sciences to understand oneself and one's relationship with other people and to comprehend the nature and function of communities.
7. Understand the physical world and interrelationship with human activity to make decisions based on scientific evidence and be responsive to individual and community values and interests.
8. Comprehend life and time from historical and contemporary perspectives and draw from past experiences to influence the present and future.
9. Gain a perspective on social, political and economic issues for resolving societal and professional problems.
10. Comprehend the meaning of human spirituality to recognize the relationship of beliefs to culture, behavior, health and healing. (AACN, 1986)
11. Appreciate the role of the fine and performing arts in stimulating individual creativity, expressing personal feelings and emotions, and building a sense of the commonality of human experience.
12. Understand the nature of human values and develop a personal philosophy to make ethical judgments in both a personal and professional life.

This document also addressed critical components for faculty of nursing programs. It identified nursing faculty as being responsible for integrating liberal arts and science knowledge into professional nursing education and practice. This

"Essentials" document has been revised in response to changes in health care over the years. The last document published to date was in 2008 and entitled *The Essentials for Baccalaureate Education for Professional Nursing Education.* This document addressed curricular elements and the framework for building the baccalaureate curriculum in nursing for the 21st century. Nine essential outcomes expected of graduates from baccalaureate programs as generalist and identified as:

Essential I:	Liberal Education for Baccalaureate Generalist Nursing Practice.
Essential II:	Basic Organizational and Systems Leadership for Quality Care and Patient Safety.
Essential III:	Scholarship for Evidence Based Practice.
Essential IV:	Information Management and Application of Patient Care Technology.
Essential V:	Health Care Policy, Finance and Regulatory Environments.
Essential VI:	Interpersonal Communication and Collaboration for Improving Patient Health Outcomes.
Essential VII:	Clinical Prevention and Population Health.
Essential VIII:	Professionalism and Professional Values.
Essential IX:	Baccalaureate Generalist Nursing Practice. (AACN, 2008)

As a result of a generalist education, baccalaureate-prepared nurses have a variety of health care settings in which they can practice at various levels from bedside or home care to administration. These nurses can serve as advocates to ensure quality health care practices and promote nursing as a profession.

Graduate Education

Graduate education can be an individual's initial degree into the nursing profession, but this is not common. Many nurses enter graduate programs following completion of a BSN and a work experience that allows them to specialize in an area of special interest. This prepares the individual for advanced practice in their area of interest.

Due to the limited graduate programs in nursing prior to 1960, many nurses desiring to obtain graduate degrees were forced to select other disciplines of interest. Most nurses in the ten-year span between 1950 and 1960 viewed the master's degree as a terminal degree for the nurse educational experience. This view of the master's degree as the final educational experience was soon overshadowed by the recognition that doctoral degrees were needed in order to place nurses on a par with other disciplines. As a result, there has been a substantial growth of graduate nursing programs.

Entry into graduate nursing programs vary, with most requiring a baccalaureate degree in nursing from an accredited program, an unencumbered nursing license (a license free of any restrictions by the state for potential sanctions), completion of an aptitude examination (e.g., Graduate Record Examination), and a designated grade point average on undergraduate study. Some programs require some work experience, but in response to encouragement to increase the numbers of advanced practice nurses, some programs permit continuation from the baccalaureate degree directly into graduate study.

Many graduate programs can be completed in 12 to 18 months of full-time study and 24 months of part-time study. Students have an option to select an area of advanced practice that could focus on adult health, pediatrics, critical care, administration, education, informatics, nurse anesthesia, nurse practitioner, or other areas of clinical specialization. The curriculum will generally include a core of courses taken by all students regardless of the specific area of study, which might include theory, research, advanced health assessment, advanced pharmacology, advanced pathophysiology, and/or other courses that are identified by the specific nursing program. Completion of graduate programs may include a research study or thesis, successful completion of a comprehensive examination, or completion of a clinically based project.

Nurses graduating from master's degree programs usually earn a master of science (MS) or a master of science in nursing (MSN) degree. Some graduate programs offer combination degrees for nurses with a non-nursing degree being earned simultaneously with one in nursing. These can include master of science in nursing/master of business administration (MSN/MBA), master of science in nursing/master of health administration (MSN/MHA), etc. These degrees are not offered by all programs. Many continue to offer a nursing degree with a single focal area.

Doctoral education in nursing began in 1910 at Teachers College, Columbia University. The degree offered was a doctor of philosophy, or PhD. This degree was and is still considered to not be specific to nursing, but rather a research degree. Graduates from these programs are expected to expand theory and conduct research. Some nurses, in an effort to focus their doctoral study in an area directed toward education, obtained the doctor of education, or EdD degree. Graduates from this program are expected to work in academia or in administration or specialized educational positions. There are still individual nurses who are enrolled in doctoral study outside of nursing, but the preference for employment in nursing education and other areas that are nursing focused is a degree that is in the discipline.

The doctor of nursing practice (DNP) is a degree focused on moving the current level of advanced nursing practice from master's preparation to doctoral level. This degree grew out of the American Association of Colleges of Nursing's (AACN) *Position Statement on the Practice Doctorate in Nursing*. This nursing doctorate (ND) was first offered at Case Western Reserve University in 1979. Prior to this time, nursing focused on research-based doctoral degrees or professional doctorates. Professional doctorates at most universities included the doctor of nursing science (DNS or DNSc). These degrees were closely aligned to the PhD in preparation of graduates. A doctoral degree that resulted from a practice-focused curriculum in nursing was offered by some programs under varying programs of study, which included nurse doctorate (ND) or doctor of nursing practice (DNP or DrNP). AACN offered 13 recommendations for a unified approach to the practice-focused doctoral program of study in their position statement:

> Recommendation 1: The term practice doctorate be used instead of clinical doctorate.
>
> Recommendation 2: The practice focused doctoral program be a distinct model of doctoral education that provides an additional option for attaining a terminal degree in the discipline.
>
> Recommendation 3: Practice-focused doctoral programs prepare graduates for the highest level of nursing practice beyond the initial preparation in the discipline.
>
> Recommendation 4: Practice-focused doctoral nursing programs include seven essential areas of content: (1) scientific underpinnings for practice, (2) advanced nursing practice, (3) organization and system leadership/management, quality improvement and system thinking, (4) analytic methodologies, (5) utilization of technology and information for health care improvement and transformation, (6) health policy development, implementation and evaluation, and (7) interdisciplinary collaboration.
>
> Recommendation 5: Practice doctoral nursing programs should include development and/or validation of expertise in at least one area of specialized advanced nursing practice.
>
> Recommendation 6: Practice-focused doctoral nursing programs prepare leaders for nursing practice and be considered the terminal practice degree.
>
> Recommendation 7: One degree title should be chosen to represent practice-focused doctoral programs.
>
> Recommendation 8: The Doctor of Nursing Practice (DNP) be the degree associated with practice-focused nursing education.
>
> Recommendation 9: The Doctor of Nursing (ND) title be phased out.
>
> Recommendation 10: The practice doctorate be the graduate degree for advanced nursing practice preparation.
>
> Recommendation 11: A transition period be planned to provide nurses with master's degrees who wish to obtain the doctoral degree a mechanism to earn a practice doctorate in a relatively streamlined fashion.
>
> Recommendation 12: Practice doctorate programs are encouraged to offer additional coursework and practica that would prepare graduates to fill the role of nurse educator.
>
> Recommendation 13: Practice-focused doctoral programs need to be accredited by a nursing accrediting agency recognized by the U.S. Secretary of Education. (AACN, 2004).

This document served to unify the approach to nursing practice doctoral programs. As of 2007, there were 53 DNP programs with that number rising. This education option has grown in popularity among nurses.

Quality and Safety Education for Nurses (QSEN)

Nursing is a profession that requires knowledge and skills in order to safely manage patient health care in various settings. In an effort to address this challenge to nursing education, the Quality and Safety Education for Nurses (QSEN) was funded by the Robert Wood Johnson Foundation in 2005. The basis of this project is to educate nursing students on patient safety issues and mechanisms to improve health care quality. This project not only addresses knowledge and skills but the attitudes necessary for the individual desiring to become a nurse. The knowledge, skills, and attitude combination is designed to promote continuous improvement in the health care setting by future nurses who will work there. QSEN promotes the use of patient-centered care, teamwork and collaboration, evidence-based practice in care delivery, quality improvement, safety, and informatics in the learning environment of the nurse. These will be reviewed below.

Patient-Centered Care

Patient-centered care promotes allowing the patient to be a full partner in their care. They have ultimate control of care activities and decisions regarding their health care activities. It is important for the nurse to be aware of the many dimensions of patient-centered care. These dimensions include knowledge of preferences in care based on interactions of the patient, family, and community in which they live, coordination of care among all providers, the need for communication and information regarding care activities and health status updates, the need for physical comfort and emotional support during their illness episodes, involvement of family as well as friends, and their transition from nurse-given care to self-care and continuity of care. Skills include the ability to perform activities that promote these dimensions and implementation of an individualized plan of care for each patient. Attitudes are important and affect care components. It is imperative that the patient be viewed with respect and their knowledge base recognized regarding their individual illness or disease process. It is important for the nurse to be self-aware and willingly support individuals whose values differ from their own.

Patient-centered care extends to comprehensive understanding of the many disease processes that result in pain and suffering, an awareness of patient empowerment aspects in health care, ethical and legal issues in patient-centered care, and collaboration and communication in promoting care. Nurses need to be astute in their assessment skills and implementation of techniques to address pain and suffering as well as removing barriers to the promotion of empowerment. Valuing active partnerships can assist in increasing patient respect and increasing active engagement of both the patient and family. The use of shared decision making can promote success in patient outcomes.

Teamwork and Collaboration

The nurse is just one member of an interdisciplinary team that interacts with patients in the delivery of care. Nurses must work collaboratively with other health care professionals in health promotion and disease prevention activities. Successful patient outcomes can depend on the attainment of this collaboration. It is important for nurses to be knowledgeable of the roles of individuals on the team. Often, roles overlap in their responsibilities in patient care management. It is important for all care providers to be able to work through clearly identifying roles and account-abilities that demonstrate recognition of the value, expertise, and perspective of each team member. This is imperative in order for the team to function cohesively in the delivery of safe care. This allows team members to initiate request for assistance that acknowledges the expertise of each team member that promotes team success in care activities and patient management.

Nurses must learn skills that promote cohesive team functioning inclusive of con-flict resolution. Conflict resolution strategies include such things as listening with respect and responding with care to breathing techniques to convey calmness and confidence. It is important to know when to assert one's own position versus support-ing that of another team member. It is important to effectively use communication styles based on the situation and personality of individuals involved. There are basi-cally three communication styles: aggressive, passive, and assertive. Becoming more self-aware and understanding one's own personal style of communication can assist in creating a good working care delivery team.

It is important for the nurse to assess their own communication strengths and weaknesses in an effort to promote improvement of this skill. Use of communication practices promoted to reduce patient risks when engaging in hand-off activities (e.g., giving a patient condition report to a nurse or other care provider who will assume care from a designated point in time for continued care or administration of specific interventions) should be followed. These improve patient outcomes and promote quality and safe care.

Evidence-Based Practice in Health Care

Evidence based knowledge is foundational to quality care delivery. Nursing has its history in borrowed knowledge from other disciplines. It is continuously working to develop a research or evidence-based environment that validates nursing activities. It is important that quality care be based on research and not opinion. Research plays a critical role in determining best patient care practices. Nurses have a responsibility to validate the strength of the evidence used for choices made regarding nursing interventions. Nurses should be able to evaluate the quality of research studies and select those that best demonstrate research processes and outcomes toward success. This is important in initial selection, continued use, or modification of best practice decisions.

Research is used in the clinical and/or classroom preparation of nurses. An appre-ciation of this information is important. Validation of care activities through the use of research is integration. The new graduate nurse is a consumer of research, using research to promote understanding and verification of care. This allows the nurse to effectively validate care activities and outcomes. Nurses at all levels must learn to value research as well as appreciate the strengths and weaknesses of this process in the delivery of care. Knowledge of how to evaluate research is an important skill, from its ethical underpinnings to its quality in methodology and results. Knowledge of the research process and how it is integral to validation of patient outcomes is foundational to the learning process. This is necessary in order to continue to improve care through use and involvement in the research process at all levels of nursing. Identifying self-limitations and the acquisition of increased knowledge regarding research and its use allows the nurse to increase their knowledge base in this area. The ultimate outcome is increased quality and safety in patient care.

Quality Improvement

Data is used to monitor outcomes and continuously improve quality and safety in health care systems. Knowledge regarding quality improvement (QI) and outcomes is important to include in the educational process. This is a continuous process in organizations, and QI affects patient safety. Students are part of the health care system and affect the overall quality of patient care. It is important for them to be familiar with tools that are used for care and evaluation of sentinel events (events that occur due to failure to adhere to pre-identified policies and procedures, e.g., patient fall). Health care is constantly changing in an effort to give safe, economical care. Effective changes need a collaborative team approach for success. Changes should be initiated based on evidence and proper change strategies are important to use in an effort to promote the change in an organization.

Safety

System effectiveness and individual performance can be used to minimize the risk of harm to patients and providers. Safety initiatives include human and safety-enhancing technologies (e.g., barcodes, medication pumps, automatic bed alarms, etc.). Knowledge and effective use of strategies are important factors in patient safety. All nurses need to know and value their role in preventing errors in promoting safe patient care. Strategies such as effective open communication can promote safety for patients and providers. Communication strategies reduce the probability of error in receiving orders and delegation of care activities. Promoting vigilance and monitoring performance of self and others can facilitate safe patient outcomes.

Informatics

Technology is the basis of many health care organizations. Applications include electronic charting to requisitions for laboratory or radiological information. Patient personal information databases in the computerized system can be readily accessed for update or verification of care activities. Knowing the legal and ethical mechanisms for management of this information is a must. There are technological benefits and limitations. Many systems are designed to initiate alerts and monitor activities related to care activities (e.g., medication removal from a computerized system will be logged into a computer database). Knowledge of technology and information management tools that support safe care initiatives are imperative. It is important to recognize the need for nurse involvement in designing, selecting, implementing, and evaluating technology-based systems in health care organizations.

Summary

The professions history has demonstrated a slow but deliberate move from hospital to higher education. There is no consensus on the entry level for nursing, although it was proposed over 30 years ago. Graduate education is on the rise, with education moving toward a practice doctorate for advanced practice entry. The doctorate is now considered the terminal degree for nursing practice. The educational pathway for nurses continues to respond to societal challenges as needs change and care becomes more complex.

References

American Association of Colleges of Nursing (2004). AACN Position Statement on the Practice Doctorate in Nursing. Retrieved from http://www.aacn.nche.edu/DNP/DNPPositionStatement.htm

American Association of Colleges of Nursing. (2008). The essentials of baccalaureate education for professional nursing practice. Washington, DC: American Association of Colleges of Nursing.

AACN (American Association of Colleges of Nursing). 1986. Essentials of College and University Education for Professional Nursing: Final Report. Washington, DC: AACN.

American Nurses Association (1965). Educational preparation for nurse practitioners and assistants to nurses, a position paper. Kansas City, MO: American Nurses Association.

Cronenwett, L., Sherwood, G., Barnsteiner J., Disch, J., Johnson, J., Mitchell, P., Sullivan, D., & Warren, J. (2007). Quality and safety education for nurses. *Nursing Outlook, 55*(3)122–131.

Institute of Medicine. (2003). Health professions education: A bridge to quality. Washington, DC: National Academies Press.

Lysaught, J. (1970). *An Abstract for Action.* New York: McGraw Hill.

National League for Nursing (2000). *Educational Competencies for Graduates of Associate Degree Nursing Programs.* New York: National League for Nursing.

National League for Nursing. (2006). A Guide to State-Approved Schools of Nursing RN, 58th ed. New York: National League for Nursing.

National League for Nursing Accrediting Commission, Inc. (2008). *NLNAC 2008 Standards and Criteria: Diploma programs in nursing.* Retrieved from http://www.nlnac.org/manuals/SC2008_DIPLOMA.htm

Quality and Safety Education for Nurses (QSEN). Funded by the Robert Wood Johnson Foundation. Retrieved from http://www.qsen.org/

U.S. Department of Health and Human Services Health Resources and Services Administration (2010). *The registered nurse population: Findings from the 2008 national survey of registered nurses.* Retrieved from http://bhpr.hrsa.gov/healthworkforce/rnsurveys/rnsurveyfinal.pdf

Chapter 12: Evidence-Based Nursing Practice

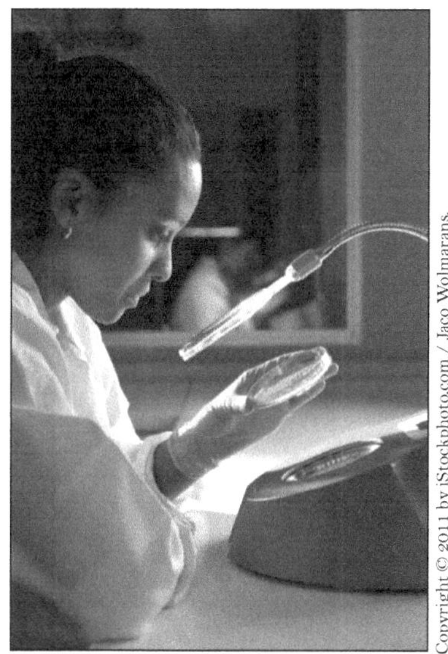

E vidence-based practice (EBP) is nursing care with a foundation in research validation for implementation. As with some other components of nursing, nursing research dates back to Florence Nightingale and her validation of observations made related to issues that significantly affected patient care and outcomes. Nursing's research history began slowly and was mainly used for education rather than validation of patient care outcomes. This was in part due to the fact that nursing was only beginning to have nurses with the educational expertise to conduct research studies. Nursing research was also not highly financially subsidized for intense research or longitudinal studies over time. But times have changed. Research has evolved to be a critical foundation for nursing practice, and this chapter will explore evidence-based practice and its link to nursing research.

Evidence-based practice (EBP) is a problem-solving method for health care delivery that integrates the best evidence from research studies to develop solutions for a health care problem. This information is further integrated with relevant patient care data, preferences, and values, and then merged with nurse expertise to develop a strategy that promotes the best health care outcome possible for a patient.

There are some basic steps to EBP. These steps include:

1. ASK—Conversion of information need into an answerable question.
2. ACQUIRE—Find the best evidence.
3. APPRAISE—Critically appraise results of literature search for validity and usefulness.
4. APPLY—Apply findings to clinical practice.
5. ASSESS—Evaluate professional performance.

Adapted from Straus, S. E., Richardson, W. S., Glasziou, P., & Haynes, R. B. (2011). *Evidence-Based Medicine: How to Practice and Teach It.* 2nd ed. London: Churchill-Livingstone, 2000:3–4. and Flemming, K. (1998). Asking answerable questions [editorial]. Evidence-based nursing; 1:36–37.

These steps will be briefly reviewed.

ASK—Conversion of information need into an answerable question is Step One. This involves formulation of a clinical question. Here the nurse needs to ask questions in a format that can be answered with specific information. It is important to define the question and structure it for the appropriate setting, as this technique is not only applicable to the clinical environment but management as well. The question may be directed to a management issue relevant to nursing. There are usually four parts to question construction: the patient/problem (P), the intervention (I), the comparison (C), and the outcome (O). The acronym for this is PICO. Using this framework for question development allows for structured follow-through for the following steps.

The four PICO elements should be evident in a well-structured question. This way you can develop a focused question that will allow for retrieval of specific research results in the next evidence-based step. If your question is too broad, you may end up with thousands of results and if it is too narrow, you may not have any results of your search. A well-formed question also allows for identification of key words to use in the "ACQUIRE" step of the EBP process. This can save a lot of valuable time during research study retrieval. Let's use a situation to develop a question using PICO.

Review this scenario: You work in a busy labor and delivery unit. Patients are admitted for a brief period of time for delivery of their newborn. All patients admitted who report "smoking during pregnancy" during history retrieval are given a brochure about quitting smoking. The nurse interacts with the mother for a very brief period of time addressing this brochure. This information is only reviewed once during the admission. You and other coworkers are concerned that these mothers will resume smoking with the new infant in the home and that the one-time brochure review is not adequate to cause cessation of smoking in the mother after discharge. You and several other nurses working on the unit decide to identify if this minimal contact and brochure review is adequate based on the available research to affect smoking. See Table 1 for use of PICO to develop the question.

Focus question result = *In hospitalized maternal patients, does a short, one-time educational nursing intervention, compared to no intervention, lead to smoking cessation?* This allows for identification of key words such as smoking cessation and education for information retrieval. This would lead to more specific studies being returned in the database.

ACQUIRE—Finding the best evidence is Step Two. This is a critical step. It is important to make sure you locate information that both supports and negates interventions. These are best located in peer-reviewed journals. These are journals where published articles are reviewed by other nurse researchers for quality and relevance before they are published in the journal. Many times the perfect article is located but there is a cost associated with retrieval. The local hospital librarian may be able to assist with retrieval at no cost. There may also be information located online, but this information must be critically reviewed for quality. Literature searches through well-known search engines may also retrieve thousands of "hits," but their relevance and quality must be reviewed individually. This can be a time-consuming endeavor.

APPRAISE—Critically appraising results of the literature search for validity and usefulness is Step Three. Critical analysis of the article type is where to begin for this step. It is important to identify only research studies or systematic analyses of the research for inclusion in the list of articles for use. Only use articles that fit the format for quantitative research, qualitative research, or a systematic review of the literature. Systematic reviews of research are articles where authors have collected numerous research studies and based on criteria for inclusion or exclusion, compared and contrasted these studies for their findings. They appraise these articles and arrive at conclusions from all of the included studies. They can be very beneficial in validating a thorough review of key research studies for certain topics of interest.

APPLY—Application of findings to clinical practice is Step Four. In this step, you integrate the evidence into practice decisions and activities. This information is combined with the unique needs and values of the patient to achieve the best outcome.

ASSESS—Evaluation of professional performance is Step Five. This allows for critical appraisal of the outcome following implementation of the EBP validated activity. Assessment should take into account the perspective of other health care providers, which can give varying perspectives and credibility to the assessment.

Table 1. Using PICO in the ASK step of EBP

P	I	C	O
Hospitalized maternal smokers	A short, one-time educational nursing intervention	No treatment	Smoking cessation (patient reported)

After identifying the fiscal efficiency and clinical effectiveness of the intervention, changes can be made to policies and procedures.

It is important to bridge the gap between the evidence and bedside use of this evidence. Nursing students should take any research course seriously, knowing that this information will be foundational to their future practice. Nursing is ever evolving and information is increasingly available. This can present an overwhelming task for review and critique related to relevance and use. There is also a current nursing shortage, which adds to the demand of nurses working with patients in various settings. These things make it difficult for nurses to engage in activities that require time and effort that some feel may distract from the importance of patient care. A balance is imperative in order to continually address nursing research topics of interest in the delivery of care that promotes the best patient outcome.

What Is Nursing Research?

Nursing research is applying scientific inquiry to a phenomenon of concern for nursing. It is to "search and search again" for an answer to this phenomenon of interest. Nurses conduct research in an effort to build a body of knowledge that is unique to nursing, validate improvements that are proposed for nursing interventions, and promote cost management in health care. Nursing research is a more formalized process than that used for EBP problem solving (see Table 2).

There can be two broad categories for research. These categories include quantitative research and qualitative research. Quantitative research uses methods that are more objective and uses techniques that allow replication or duplication of the research study. This type of research is more based on the retrieval of numbers or data that can be counted or measured with standardized instruments or questionnaires. Statistical techniques are used that allow quantification and numerical differentiation or similarity identification. Quantitative research is deductive in its approach.

Table 2. Comparison of Steps in the EBP Problem-Solving Process and the Research Process

Evidence-Based Practice Problem Solving Process	Research Process
1. ASK—Conversion of information need into an answerable question.	1. Identify a research topic.
2. ACQUIRE—Find the best evidence.	2. Review the literature to identify what is already known.
3. APPRAISE—Critically appraise results of literature search for validity and usefulness.	3. Define the research purpose and formulate questions or hypotheses.
No comparative step.	4. Select the research design.
No comparative step.	5. Select the sample or population.
No comparative step.	6. Collect study data.
4. APPLY—Apply findings to clinical practice.	7. Analyze study data to generate conclusions and implications.
5. ASSESS—Evaluate professional performance.	
No comparative step.	8. Communicate study results.

Deductive approaches move from a general case, which in research is identifying a research question or hypothesis, to a specific instance or precise measurements and analyses. Qualitative research uses methods that are more subjective in their approach. This approach uses methods of inquiry that emphasizes retrieval of the meaning of the experience for a given individual. The researcher is an integral part of this process. They may conduct or work with others to conduct interviews or methods of verbal interaction, which are often used to obtain data from subjects involved in the study. Researchers reduce these words to themes (single words or phrases) that evolve from critical analyses of words retrieved through the data collection process. Qualitative research is inductive in its approach. Inductive approaches move from specific situations, which are the interviews of individuals who address the common topic of the research (e.g., to broader generalizations or themes (specific topics) derived from the numerous interviews. See Box 1 for examples of the two general types of research.

Box 1. Example of Types of Research

Quantitative Research Abstract

Tinne Dilles, Robert Vander Stichele, Bart Van Rompaey, Lucas Van Bortel & Monique Elseviers, "Nurses' Practices in Pharmacotherapy and their Association with Educational Level (Abstract)," *Journal of Advanced Nursing*, vol. 66, no. 5. Copyright © 2010 by John Wiley & Sons, Inc. Reprinted with permission.

Abstract

Title. Nurses' practices in pharmacotherapy and their association with educational level.

Aim. This paper is a report of a study of the association between educational level and nurses' practices in pharmacotherapeutic activities in three clinical settings.

Background. The preparation and administration of medication are at the core of nursing practice, and nurses' involvement in pharmacotherapy is essential to medication safety. Nursing strategies to improve patient adherence to treatment and to identify adverse drug reactions have been described, but nurses' practice patterns in monitoring adherence and adverse drug reactions remain undocumented.

Methods. A cross-sectional correlational survey design was used. Data were collected between 2005 and 2007. Each year, the focus was on a different setting. Nurses were selected by convenience sampling: 260 worked in nursing homes, 82 in community care services and 1070 in hospitals. Questions focused on the provision of medication information, observation of patient medication adherence and identification of adverse drug reactions during the preceding month.

Results. Involvement in providing drug information varied considerably, from 50% among hospital nurses to 82% among nurses in community care services. Statistically significantly fewer nurses observed non-adherence in hospitals (50%) than in the other settings (about 80%). Between 40% and 49% of the nurses had observed an adverse drug reaction. Nurses' information-seeking behaviour and problem responses also varied according to setting. Bachelor's degree holders were 35% more likely than diploma holders to have observed an adverse drug reaction.

Conclusion. Nurses assume considerable pharmacotherapeutic responsibilities. Practice patterns are codetermined by the healthcare setting and nurses' educational level.

Qualitative Research Abstract

Peterson, J., Johnson, M., Halvorsen, B., Apmann, L., Chang, P., Kershek, S., & Pincon, D. (2010). Where do nurses go for help? A qualitative study of coping with death and dying. *International Journal of Palliative Nursing*, 16(9), 432–438.

Abstract

Title. Where do nurses go for help? A qualitative study of coping with death and dying.

Aim. This paper is a report of a study aimed at identifying how nurses cope with death and dying in their patient contacts and the resources they use in coping with loss.

Background. Nurses are individuals who may develop relationships with patients due to the frequency of contact. Patient interactions have been reported to be a very fulfilling aspect of the nursing profession. Due to this relationship nurses can experience stress associated with patient death.

Methods. A qualitative grounded theory approach was used in this research study. Audiotaped in-depth interviews and online open ended surveys were used to collect data regarding experiences of nurses and nursing students who cared for dying patients. Fifteen nurses and nursing students participated. Data was transcribed and verified.

Results. Nurses in the study reported several mechanisms they used for coping with patient death. These strategies relied on internal and external sources. Themes for internal sources that emerged included evaluating death (looking at death as part of life) and relying on professional distance. Themes from external sources that emerged included looking to peers for support and advice, religious resources including their own beliefs, and the patients and families themselves for comfort.

Conclusion. End of life is becoming a prominent issue in healthcare. In order to successfully cope with the stress of caring for a dying patient, nurses need programs that facilitate coping with this experience.

Research is a validated way of knowing for nursing. Prior to a more extensive use of research to validate many interventions, the nursing profession retrieved knowledge through traditions, authority, borrowing, trial and error, personal experience, role modeling and intuition. Use of reasoning and research are foundational to delivery of care for nurses in the current evidence-based environment. Research uses a process to promote retrieval and dissemination of study results in order to achieve the best patient outcomes. Many questions or topics of interest arrive from the nurse's clinical practice. Some may also result from reading the research of others or course work for advanced practice study (see Figure 1).

Research is now a driving force in nursing. Nurses at all education levels have a place in the research process. Nurses at the bedside are pivotal in identifying problems and collecting for analyses. This serves to expand the base of nursing research. Expanding the research base for nursing also expands the amount of evidence available for use to manage patient care situations.

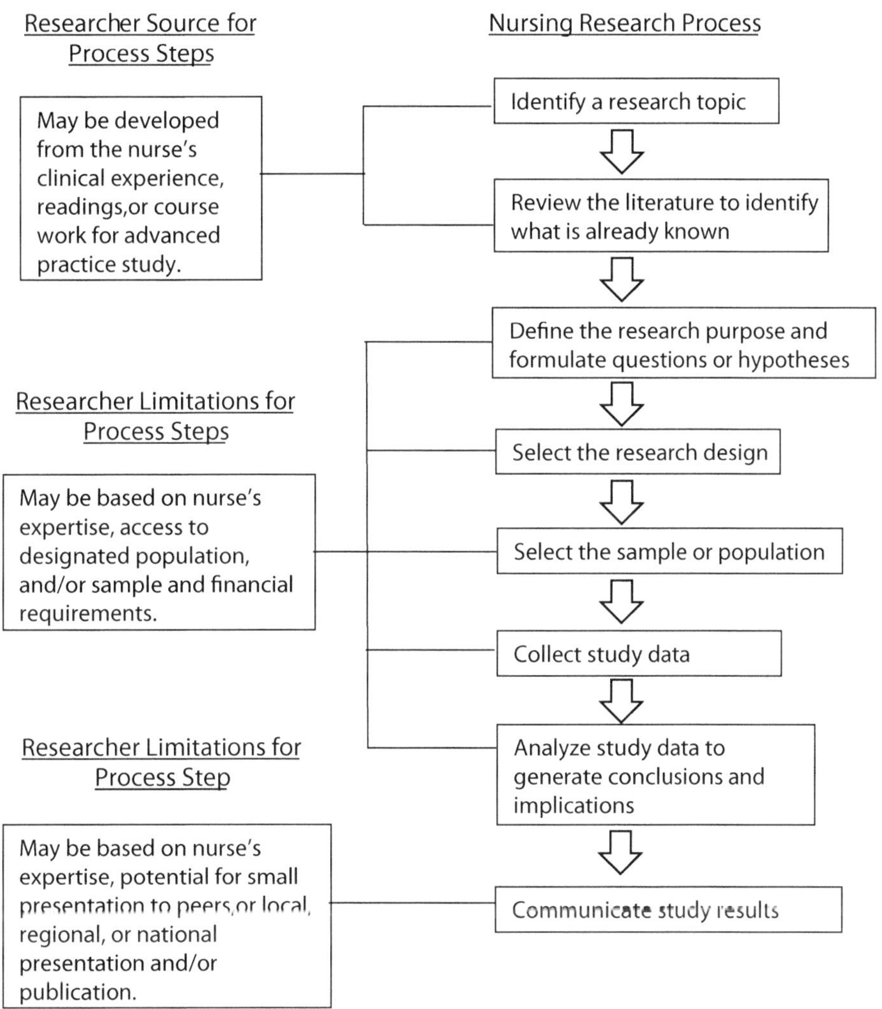

Figure 1. Stages of the Research Process with Researcher Source or Limitations

The Research Process

Research allows movement of information from an abstract idea to the realities of knowing. It allows a researcher to test or validate responses or answer questions posed through clinical experiences or other situations. This section is intended to give you a brief introductory review to the research process in order to prompt interest and a desire to learn more. It is not comprehensive, as research is a process with many sub-activities that must be completed in order to comply with regulations for initiation of the research process and ultimate success of the project. Quantitative and qualitative research processes are not the same, but the following steps can be adjusted for either form of research.

Research is systematic inquiry. It requires adherence to a specific format for investigation in order to have results that meet criteria for scientific merit. Collaborative research is a good place to start when looking to get involved in research. This allows you to learn while doing and establishes a peer mentoring relationship that can be mutually beneficial. Use of textbooks and other material that assists with specifics of the research process, including statistical analyses, is also beneficial. Give the process enough time to allow for success. Do not expect to complete this process in a few days. A brief review of steps in the research process is identified below.

Identify the Research Topic

This is a global step that allows for identification of an area of interest in order to generate a specific question. This area of interest may result from any activity that stimulates why, when, what, how, etc. questions on topics related to an activity that could lead to a specific outcome. Questions resulting from these topics can be expanded to specifically address areas. You want to make sure that the question is asked in such a way that guides you forward in the process. This step may appear as follows. General area of interest one—ventilator-associated pneumonia. This has resulted from the fact that in the past 30 days out of 12 ventilator-dependent patients, eight of them have acquired pneumonia and required extensive additional care, causing patient and family distress. Let's look at another one. General area of interest two—readmission of patients diagnosed with congestive heart failure (CHF). Over the past three months, six of the nine patients diagnosed with CHF have been readmitted within 30 days of discharge due to eating foods high in sodium (salt) or not adhering to their medication regimen (taking medications as prescribed). General area of interest three—asthma in children. Asthma is a very common childhood disease that affects quality of life for children. You work in a pediatrician's office where children appear to be disinterested in the current asthma care program. You are interested in developing a program that is of interest to these children with asthma in an effort to promote quality of life.

Review the Literature to Identify What Is Already Known

Now you need to see what others had to say about your specific area of research interest. You need to know if there are similar studies to support your research topic. You do this by looking in the research literature to identify what research has been done in the past by individuals interested in these topics. This is the literature review. You may find a completed supporting study that you can replicate for your specific area. All of the literature review news may not be good news. You may also find that the literature does not support your original thought or question. It has been thoroughly investigated in the research and found to be detrimental to patient outcomes. This will require you to rethink and restructure your research study.

The literature review is a critical part of defining the research process. Give preference to literature that is current or within the past five years. This step usually requires a significant outlay of time and effort. This is where a collaborative effort may be very helpful. If you have a peer in an advanced educational nursing program looking to do a project for a specific course, this may be an ideal way to get some much needed assistance to retrieve and critique research as well as help with the entire research process. A relationship involving this person in the research study may be mutually beneficial.

When performing the literature review, be sure to keep notes on what has been retrieved. Keep a log of key words used in searches to prevent duplication of this work. Use databases that will give you access to research-based articles and not just general information articles. Look for articles that are in peer-reviewed journals. This means that the articles have been evaluated by a group of peer nurse researchers for quality and relevance. They also evaluate their adherence to the research process. Identify specific search categories to reduce retrieved relevant articles to a manageable number. When you come across an article that you think might be useful, immediately retrieve it for later reference. This can save you significant time later in searching for "that article I saw two days ago that would be perfect."

One mechanism to use to validate an exhaustive literature review is to critically analyze the reference list of appropriate research studies. These can give you a lot of information regarding other relevant research on your topic. Once you start to see duplication of research in the reference lists and do not identify new articles in these lists compared to your own list of articles reviewed, you know that your literature review phase has come to a close. Articles that review research literature on the topic can save you time critiquing articles for relevance. These are called systematic reviews of the literature, and can be an excellent source of information regarding types of research on your topic along with study quality.

Define the Research Purpose

Your next move is defining the purpose. Leaving the topic general can be overwhelming and not allow you to address what you are really interested in finding out. What do you really want to know? What question will allow you to address specific areas of true interest? Looking at the area of general interest one above, you might develop a question that addresses prevention of ventilator acquired pneumonia. The question may appear as: "What is the best way to prevent ventilator associated pneumonia in my pulmonary care unit?" Looking at general area of interest two above, you might develop a question that addresses readmission of CHF patients. The question may appear as: "Does the educational intervention we are giving patients with congestive heart failure make a difference in readmission rates for these patients?" Looking at general interest area three, you might develop a question that is directed at obtaining the perspective of children between the ages of seven and ten years of age with asthma about what they see as important to include in an educational program. The question may appear as: "How do children describe their asthma experience, and based on this what do they want to know about caring for themselves?"

Select the Research Design

Now you need to select the research design. The design is the study blueprint. Here you will identify if you are going to complete a quantitative research study or qualitative research study. This will guide selection of individuals for the study and the data collection tools. This step can be affected by the nurse's level of expertise, access to the designated population, and/or sample and financial requirements (costs associated with data collection tools, paid time off to complete the research process, and/or costs required for statistical analyses).

There are many other components to consider in this phase, but for the sake of simplicity, this is the only component presented in this textbook. It is recommended that you consult a formal research textbook for specifics regarding this phase of the research project. This will identify how you progress to identifying tools needed for the research study. This detailed textbook can assist you in identification of questionnaires as well as the format for data collection.

Select the Sample or Population

This involves identifying specific individuals who will be solicited to participate in the study. This may be governed by access and permissions, which are part of the required review by a committee called an Institutional Review Board. An Institutional Review Board (IRB) is an independent ethics committee established by organizations to protect the rights of individuals being solicited for the study (called subjects). These rights and explanations are in Table 3.

A population is defined as all elements that meet designated criteria for inclusion in your study. This number can be extremely large and costly to incorporate. Your

Table 3. Individual Rights in Research

Research Right	Explanation
Right to Self-Determination	This right is based on the ethical principle of respect for others. This means that subjects should have the right to determine if they desire to participate in a study. Special considerations are made for individuals who are (a) legally or mentally incompetent;, (b) under the age of 18 years (neonates, children and teenagers); (c) have diminished capacity (e.g., mentally ill, or have a disease process that impairs their cognitive abilities like Alzheimer's disease, in a coma); (d) or are confined to an institution (e.g., mental hospital, prison).
Right to Privacy	This right means that an individual can determine the circumstances for disclosure or sharing of personal information with other people.
Right to Autonomy and Confidentiality	Autonomy means that subject identity cannot be linked to any information in the study. Confidentiality means that the researcher responsibly manages data and protects private information shared by subjects.
Right to Fair Treatment	This right is based on the ethical principle of justice, which states that each individual should have fair treatment and receive what they are due or owed.
Right to Protection from Discomfort and Harm	This right is based on the ethical principle of beneficence, which states that an individual should do good, and above all do no harm to subjects in the research study.

study may use a sample, which is a subset of the entire study population. All permissions and consents are required to be obtained prior to any data collection.

Collect Study Data

Collection of study data involves interaction of the researcher with subjects in order to collect information through observations, interviews, or completion of specific hard copy or electronic questionnaires. Study assistants may be solicited to collect study data if there is a large number of subjects to be approached and solicited for retrieval of information or if individuals are located outside the immediate area of the researcher. It is important that all individuals collecting data are familiar with the study. They should be given specific information on how to collect information, and this knowledge base verified for accuracy of the data collection process and actual data retrieved. Inaccurate data collection can affect study results and ultimately lead to invalid results. Data collectors must be familiar with the rights of study subjects and adhere to protocols to protect these rights.

Analyze Study Data

This involves differentiation of the data, data entry, and analyses. Measurement strategies in the data collection step are used to find an answer to the questions and/or hypotheses posed earlier in the process. This can appear to be an overwhelming task. It is important to perform the correct statistical tests, or the study will not be valid. Results will not represent accurate outcomes from data collected, and the research study will not present "true" results in answering or responding to initial questions or hypotheses. If you have a collaborative team of individuals, a statistician may be among them. This individual can help with quantitative research analyses. If you are doing qualitative research, you will need someone skilled in this type of data analysis. In qualitative research, there can be thousands of words to analyze and reduce to themes from subjects interviewed for data retrieval. It is important to solicit assistance and use experts to assist in determining numerical outcomes in quantitative research or themes from analysis of words collected in qualitative research.

Analyses of research findings allow for identification of study conclusions. Study findings are discussed, and information is presented to show how these findings build on and add to the body of knowledge identified in the review of the literature. This allows for identification of whether the study supports or does not support previous research findings. This area will also allow the discussion of implications and relevance to clinical practice. Specific contributions to the body of knowledge can be presented along with areas for future research on the topic.

Communicate Study Results

Communicating your results is the final step in the research process. This allows others access to your research for use in evidence-based practice for care delivery to patients, families, and communities. A research report will be written and appropriate venues identified for dissemination of study findings. This may be on a local, regional, national, or international level. It may involve publishing information in journals that may be in hard-copy or electronic format. It is important to communicate findings in an effort to build the body of nursing knowledge.

Research Organizations in Nursing

National Nursing Research Organizations

National Institute of Nursing Research. The National Institute of Nursing Research (NINR) was originally authorized through Public Law 99-158, the Health Research Extension Act of 1985, as the National Center for Nursing Research (NCNR) at the National Institute of Health (NIH) following a presidential veto override by Congress. The NCNR was officially established in 1986 with Dr. Doris Merritt, a research physician, appointed as the acting head. She served until Dr. Ada Sue Hinshaw was appointed the first nursing director. The NCNR not only supported research initiatives but supported research training and career development in health promotion and disease prevention, acute and chronic illness, and nursing systems. The center also supported strategies to improve patient outcomes. Through research training grants, beginning and advanced nurse researchers engaged in predoctoral, postdoctoral, and senior fellowships to increase individuals prepared to engage in research activities.

In 1992, following an initiative by various nursing organizations and with the support of Congress and the Executive Branch, the NIH Revitalization Act of 1993 created the NINR. The NINR has as its mission

> To promote and improve the health of individuals, families, communities, and populations. NINR supports and conducts clinical and basic research and research training on health and illness across the lifespan. The research focus encompasses health promotion and disease prevention, quality of life, health disparities, and end-of-life. NINR seeks to extend nursing science by integrating the biological and behavioral sciences, employing new technologies to research questions, improving research methods, and developing the scientists of the future. From NINR Mission. Retrieved from http://www.ninr.nih.gov/NR/rdonlyres/E54A777C-FAAA-474A-BDFF-5B85EC8B9E7E/0/StrategicMission.pdf

In promoting the mission, NINR supports clinical and basic research training on health and illness across the lifespan. Its areas of research emphasis, based on the

NINR Strategic Plan released in 2006, include health promotion and disease prevention, improving quality of life for individuals, eliminating health disparities, and end of life. Through NINR support, research in nursing has increased, and recognition achieved and promoted to the public through press releases. The Internet has also given nursing research a boost with an avenue for nurse researchers to communicate and disseminate findings on a worldwide scale.

The Council for the Advancement of Nursing Science (CANS). The American Nurses Association (ANA) restructured and disbanded the Council of Nurse Research in the late 1990's. Members quickly recognized the need to create a national nursing research-based organization. As a result, the council established CANS as an open membership entity of the American Academy of Nursing (AAN). This national organization strives to be recognized as a collective national voice for nursing science. The mission of CANS is to foster better health through nursing science. In order to accomplish this mission, the organization serves as a strong voice for nursing science on both the national and international levels. Goals are accomplished by developing, conducting, and utilizing nursing science, disseminating research findings, and facilitating lifelong learning opportunities for nurse scientists. The organization facilitates research through seed money grants, which can be up to $25,000 for organizational initiatives. Organization-specific information can be retrieved from http://www. nursingscience.org.

Regional Nursing Research Institutes/Societies

Several regional organizations exist in the United States to promote nursing research that impacts the profession of nursing and overall patient health and outcomes (see Figure 2).

These organizations were established between 1975 and 1986. They promote research on special topics based on organizationally identified research initiatives. Many offer journals to disseminate research and encourage collaborative interactions. They also offer financial support on topics of special interest to the organization. Member communication is further augmented electronically. All have online web-based information sites that are identified, along with specific information below. They are presented in the order they were established.

Midwest Nursing Research Society (MNRS). The Midwest Nursing Research Society was established in 1975 by a group of nurses working on a research project entitled the "Nursing Faculty Research Development in the Midwest." This research project was for the Department of Health and Human Services (HHS), the government's principal agency for protection of the health of U.S. citizens and provider of essential human services. During this collaborative research-based activity, these nurses discussed the need for a specific organization dedicated to nursing research. With continued effort, these initial communications formed this research-based organization. MNRS membership is drawn from nurses and nursing students living in Illinois, Indiana, Iowa, Kansas, Michigan, Minnesota, Missouri, Nebraska, North

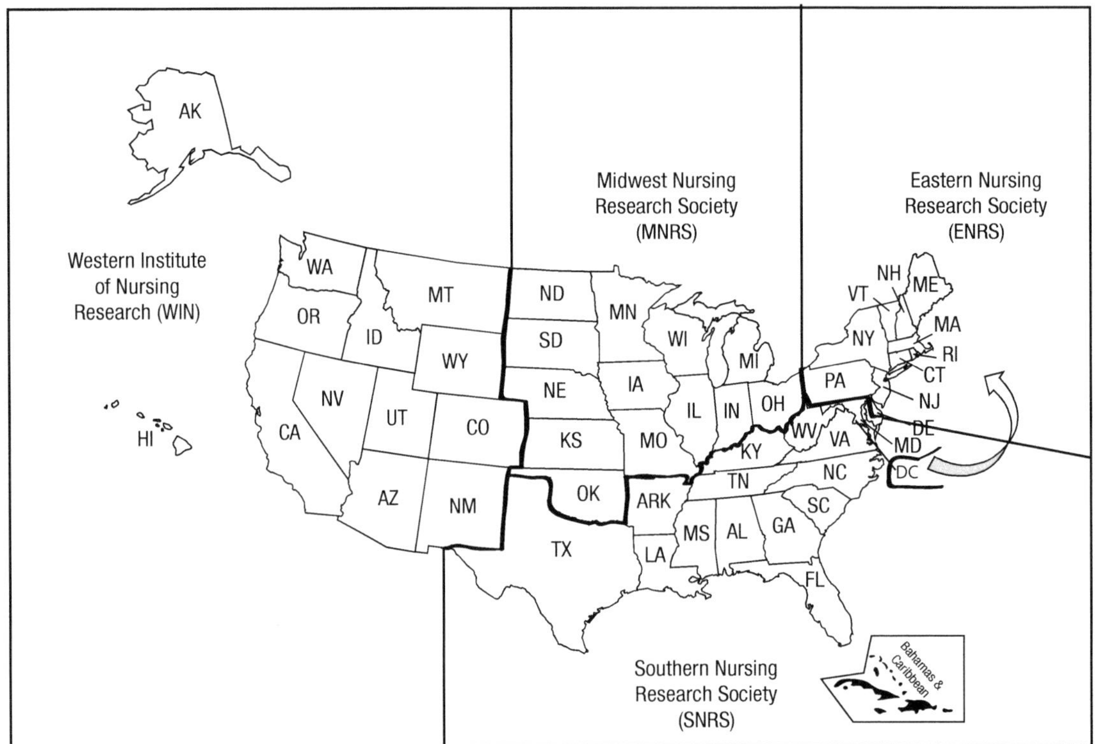

Figure 2. Regional Nursing Research Organizations

Dakota, South Dakota, Ohio, Oklahoma, and Wisconsin. The MNRS offers numerous grant opportunities that include mentorship grants, dissertation research grants, seed and new investigator grants, and others. Research areas include a multitude of topics (e.g., acute care, family health, nursing education, nursing informatics, pediatric nursing, women's health, etc.). A complete list of research topics and specifics regarding the organization's research can be obtained from http://www.mnrs.org/files/public/MNRSReseachSectionHandbook.pdf. Specific information regarding current initiatives can be obtained from the organization's website, located at http://www.mnrs.org.

Western Institute of Nursing Research (WIN). The Western Institute of Nursing Research (WIN) is a western regional nursing research organization that was formed in 1985. This organization succeeded formation of the Western Council on Higher Education for Nursing (WCHEN) following deliberation by special committees to create a research-based, autonomous, self-supporting organization. WIN consist of 13 states: Alaska, Arizona, California, Colorado, Hawaii, Idaho, Montana, Nevada, New Mexico, Oregon, Utah, Washington, and Wyoming.

WIN supports research that advances the nursing profession and improvements in practice, outcomes, and cost in health care. It supports a diverse community of nurses in their research initiatives. This organization supports research through forums for the exchange of scholarship and research, funding initiatives that support research, promotion of research in nursing education, and working with nursing research, education, and practice specialty organizations to assure a voice in health care policy for the western region of the United States. These support initiatives are further supported in organizational goals. Additional organization information can be obtained from http://www.winursing.org/.

Southern Nursing Research Society (SNRS). The Southern Nursing Research Society (SNRS) was founded in 1986 by a group of 60 nurses who collaborated to establish an organization for nursing researchers in the southern region of the United States. SNRS was officially identified as an independent organization in 1987. The original organizational membership of 14 states (Alabama, Arkansas, Florida, Georgia, Kentucky, Louisiana, Maryland, Mississippi, North Carolina, South Carolina, Tennessee, Texas, Virginia, and West Virginia) was expanded in 1991 to include the Caribbean, Latin America, and the Bahamas. SNRS has an organizational vision that values connection, collaboration, and communication among members of the research community for these states, as well as the Bahamas and countries of the Caribbean and Latin America. An annual conference allows dissemination of research for this organization. Research interest group topics allow discussion and collaborative research initiatives by individual members through the organization. Some special interest groups include aging/gerontology, education, evidence-based practice, minority health, psychiatric/mental health, and others. A listing of all special interest research groups can be located at http://snrs.org/research/research_int_groups. html. One strategic research initiative includes development of strategies to recognize and promote nursing as a science-based discipline, as well as expanding nurse researcher exposure among the general public. Additional organization information can be obtained from http://www.snrs.org

Eastern Nursing Research Society (ENRS). The Eastern Nursing Research Society (ENRS) was established in 1988 as the research arm of two existing organizations: the Mid-Atlantic Regional Nursing Association (MARNA) and the New England Organization for Nursing (NEON). The purpose of this organization was to create a community for nurses interested in research in the eastern region of the United States. This organization includes ten states (Connecticut, Delaware, Maine, Massachusetts, New Hampshire, New Jersey, New York, Pennsylvania, Rhode Island, and Vermont) and Washington, D.C. Goals of the organization include providing a networking forum for nurse scientists through conferences and online interest groups, developing nursing science, translating evidence to guide nursing practice and education as well as influence policy in these areas, and mentor nurse scientists. The organization has established research interest groups on aging; bio-behavioral issues; chronic comorbid conditions; comprehensive systematic review and knowledge translation; criminal justice, trauma and violence; family- and community-based participatory research, student research mentoring; nursing research in clinical settings; qualitative research and theory development with designated facilitators. Additional organization information can be obtained from http://www.enrs-go.org/.

Specialty Nursing Organizations

Specialty organizations are numerous in nursing. These range from academies to associations and societies in areas such as medical surgical nursing, critical care nursing, gerontological nursing, rehabilitation nursing, emergency care, long-term care, and many more (see a current listing at http://www.nurse.org/orgs.shtml). Many have research as part of their organization's mission and/or goal. They may set research-based initiatives or priorities that identify research topics of interest to the organization. Some have funds that range from a few hundred to several thousand dollars that may be obtained through an application process. These grants may be available on an annual basis. They may allow several years of research in order to address the topic of interest and allow for data collection, analysis, and dissemination of the results. Many of these organizations promote research of specialty initiatives, based on their health care focus, that increase evidence validation for clinical patient management.

Summary

The abilities to critically analyze, use, and conduct research are becoming key skills for individuals in nursing practice. Use of research promotes high-quality care provision for patients. Use of EBP in practice gives nursing a professional base of support. It is important to continue the quest to research those specific nursing issues that are important to the development of care modalities and promote the best patient outcomes. As health care changes, it is important for nurses to respond with current management that is systematic and based on empirical and observable evidence.

References

Burns, N., & Grove, S. K. (2009). *The Practice of Nursing Research: Appraisal, Synthesis, and Generation of Evidence* (6th ed.). St. Louis, MO: Elsevier Saunders.

Cope, D. (2003). Evidence-based practice: Making it happen in your clinical setting. *Clin J Oncol Nurs.* 7(1): 97–98.

Eastern Nursing Research Society at http://www.enrs-go.org/

Flemming, K. (1998). Asking answerable questions [editorial]. Evidence-based nursing; 1:36–37.

Midwest Nursing Research Society at http://www.mnrs.org/

National Institute of Nursing Research at http://www.ninr.nih.gov/

Southern Nursing Research Society at http://snrs.org

Straus, S. E., Richardson, W. S., Glasziou, P., & Haynes, R. B. (2011). *Evidence-Based Medicine: How to Practice and Teach It.* 2nd ed. London: Churchill-Livingstone, 2000:3–4.

Western Institute of Nursing Research at http://www.winursing.org/

Winsett, R., & Cashion, A. (2007). The nursing research process. *Nephrology Nursing Journal,* 34(6), 635–643.

Chapter 13: I Am a Nurse

Transitioning to the Profession

Introduction

"My job as a nurse is hard but extremely rewarding. It requires that I physically and emotionally support patients and families in my care. I must have a base of knowledge that is continually challenged and requires that I remain ever vigilant about new innovations in patient care delivery. I feel like I am always learning in order to teach my patients and peers. I truly love my patients and thoroughly enjoy helping them work to achieve a good quality of life. They hold a special place in my heart. They are the reason I love what I do. They are the reason I am a nurse."

These words spoken by one nurse relay the fundamental reasons why many individuals choose nursing as a profession. The nursing profession supports a caring attitude in administering care activities, and at its core promotes working with people to improve their health.

Transitioning from Classroom to Job

New Graduate Status

Following graduation from an accredited nursing program, you still are not allowed to use the initials RN—not even on the mortarboard (cap) at the graduation ceremony! These initials are only authorized after successfully passing a licensure examination. Following graduation, you move from studying for course grades to continuing a study regimen to be successful on the National Council Licensure Examination for Registered Nurses (NCLEX-RN). This will give you the right to use the abbreviation RN following your name. Your signature line in validating orders or notes would be your name followed by RN. Some organizations encourage you to include your terminal degree or educational preparation initials as well. The proper format would be: name (first initial and last name), degree conferred, and licensure. This would translate to the following example: B. Smith, BSN, RN. As you progress to include certifications, these can be added to your standard signature format, and the certification would follow your RN initial. Be sure to check the organization to validate the format for proper initials to use for this purpose. Movement into a management-type position may require that you alter your signature to include more information. You may also need business cards with specific information. Always comply with the regulations of the organization, but for presentations or publications, you might use this format: name (first initial and last name), degree conferred, licensure, certification, and job title. This would translate to the following: B. Smith, BSN, RN, CCRN, Clinical Nurse Manager for SICU. Be sure to check with the specific organization to identify proper signature format (whether or not to use your degree conferred and the official citation for any position). This information is generally disclosed during orientation periods. If you are using an electronic signature, this may be set and linked to your computer sign-on code so there is no need to add any additional identifiable information to notes or comments entered via the computer terminal.

Often, graduates will ask when they can wear their pin purchased from their school or college of nursing. The pin can be worn while working as a new graduate nurse. The pin symbolizes graduation from an academic institution, not licensure.

Preparing for Licensure

Upon graduation from an academic institution, the graduate nurse has successfully completed a program of academic study and earned a degree but is still not licensed to practice as a registered nurse (RN). The initials RN cannot be used until the licensure examination called the National Council Licensure Examination for Registered Nurses (NCLEX-RN) has been successfully passed. It is important to successfully navigate the examination process from preparation to completion. Preparation for the examination requires application to test in the state of initial practice. An Authorization to Test (ATT) is required and can be obtained through application to the board of nursing. Candidate eligibility to test must be declared by the board of nursing. Following this declaration, an ATT letter will be received by the candidate. This letter is required in order to schedule an appointment to take the NCLEX and enter the examination site. Each ATT letter is valid for a specific period of time and the examination must be taken within this timeframe. When presenting to the examination site, the ATT letter is to be presented, as well as an acceptable form of identification for verification (see Box 1).

It is important to prepare for the NCLEX-RN. Preparation may include self, group, and/or formal study scenarios. Self and group study sessions afford structured preparation for taking the computerized licensure examination. A formal review course may be taken in an effort to retrieve intense concentrated review time. Formal review courses are not a requirement to take the examination and should be viewed as a point of decision for the nurse candidate. Just as for any examination, arrive early, eat a good breakfast following a good night's sleep, and dress comfortably. Usually dressing in layers will allow more flexibility in adjusting body temperature. Outside

Box 1. Acceptable Forms of Identification for U.S. Test Centers

- U.S. driver's license (Department of Motor Vehicle-issued)(if expired, a renewal slip including a photograph and a signature must be presented in order to be admitted)
- U.S. state identification (Department of Motor Vehicle-issued)
- Passport
- U.S. Military Identification

From National Council of State Boards of Nursing. Acceptable identification. Retrieved from https://www.ncsbn.org/1221.htm

materials cannot be used during the testing session, but the opportunity to make notes will be available onscreen as well as access to a calculator if needed. Biometrics will also be retrieved prior to testing which may include signature, photograph, palm vein scan, and fingerprint.

The NCLEX test is offered in a computer adaptive (CAT) format. This means that the computer will vary test item difficulty around a baseline required passing score. When an item is answered incorrectly, the computer will pose an easier next item, and if an item is answered correctly, the computer will post a more difficult item for the next question. The first item is below the required passing baseline. There is a maximum testing period of five hours, but there is no time limit for each test item. Items may be in multiple choice format or alternative item format. Alternative item format may include multiple response items, fill-in-the-blank, chart/exhibit, and drag and drop. There is no designated number of alternate format items that may appear during the test. They may randomly appear at any point. Any format can include the use of charts, tables, or graphs. A test plan for the NCLEX-RN is posted to the National Council of State Boards of Nursing (NCSBN) website at https://www.ncsbn.org/1287.htm.

Seeking Employment: The Interview

Seeking employment is always a challenge for many nurses, as this is the first time they have been interviewed for a position. Nursing school offers a unique opportunity that is not afforded to other academic programs. While in clinical locations, students may identify a specific organization they are truly interested in as a first work experience following graduation. Demonstration of skill level and the ability to eagerly learn can identify individuals that may be sought out by organizations looking to hire new graduates with these traits. The formal interview will often not take place until the program of study has been completed. When seeking employment, use common-sense skills and courtesies. See interview tips in Table 1.

Modify the above tips for phone- or computer-based interviews. These are just as important and carry the same potential outcome. Be sure to get information to individuals conducting the interview in a timely manner, regardless of format.

Table 1. Interview Tips

Tip	Successful Interview Techniques
1. Prepare for the Interview	• Have a professionally prepared résumé. • Practice for the interview—this is like any other skill and takes rehearsal and repetition. • Know the organization—investigate the mission, philosophy, and goals as well as other information that can relate to the foundation for working at the organization (e.g., annual report). • Know the interview time frame and format.
2. Dress for a successful outcome.	• This is the first visual impression. • Dress professionally: • For men, this could include a solid color suit (usually black or navy) with a white or coordinated shirt, conservative shoes, limited jewelry and use of aftershave, professional hairstyle, portfolio, or briefcase. See Figure 1. • For women, this could include a solid color suit (usually black or navy) with a skirt that allows comfortable and discreet seating with a coordinated blouse, conservative shoes, limited jewelry, professional hairstyle, light make-up and perfume, and portfolio or briefcase. See Figure 2.
3. Leave early enough to arrive on time.	• Know your method of transportation. • Car travel—address any issues at least 24 hours prior to the time proposed to leave for the interview (e.g., low gasoline, engine issues, etc.). • Bus travel—know route times and potential transfers. • Taxi travel—contact the taxi company in advance to identify proper time for pick-up in order to arrive on time. • Know the route and identify potential times that have heavy traffic which can impede travel.
4. Stay calm.	• Take a deep breath prior to entering the interview room. • Remain as calm as possible during the interview. • Ask for clarification if necessary in order to address the specific question asked. • Take a moment or two to frame your response before speaking. • Fully address questions.
5. Use a handshake that relays confidence and authority.	• Should be firm but not viselike. • Stand firmly on two feet and upright when shaking hands. • If a hand is extended while seated, stand and move into the handshake.
6. Professionally present yourself.	• Carry a professional portfolio that contains information. • Use business cards to identify yourself for future contact. • Take extra copies of your résumé to the interview.
7. Take the time to say thank you upon exiting.	• Verbally thank the interviewer. • Use a follow-up thank you letter to address any issues and concerns that may have come up during the interview.

The Portfolio

Like other professionals, nurses need evidence of their growth and achievements over time, which includes the college years. The professional portfolio is a method of collecting and presenting this evidence. You need to carefully select your best work over time and use this to demonstrate how much you have learned and done in the profession. The portfolio allows reflection on one's professional life and encourages active engagement in purposeful decisions regarding growth and achievements.

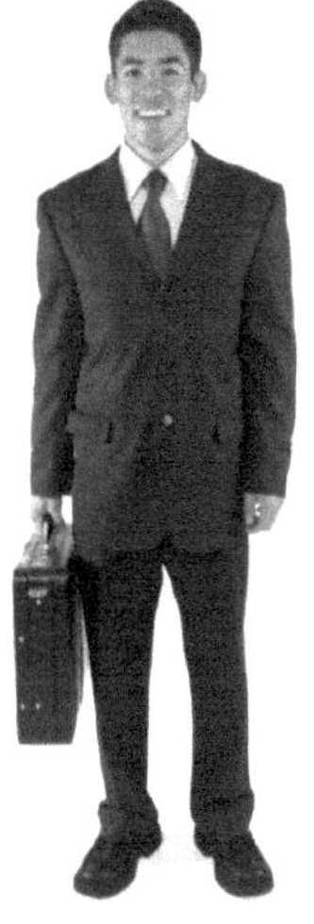

Figure 1. Dressing for a Successful Interview Outcome—Male

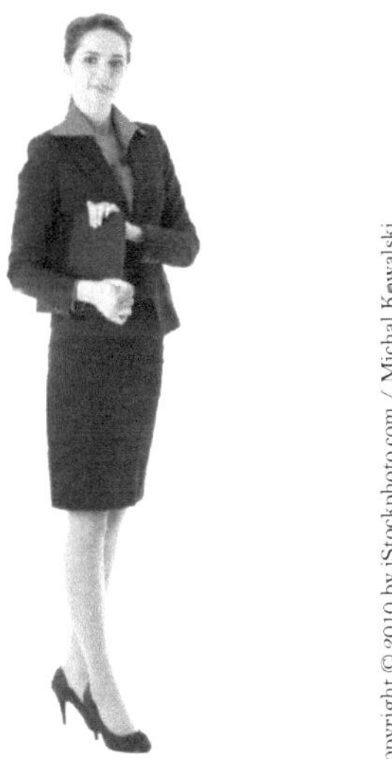

Figure 2. Dressing for a Successful Interview Outcome—Female

The Portfolio Process

The portfolio is a tool that showcases your professional work and gives evidence of career growth. It should not be something simply thrown together, but rather a purposefully crafted document. It must be meticulously constructed and demonstrate a relationship between information collection, selection, and reflection.

Box 2. Brief Outline

I. Baseline Data
- A. Why I want to be a nurse
- B. People or experiences that inspired me to enter the profession
- C. Short-Term Goals (2–4 years)
- D. Long-Term Goals (5–10 years)
- E. Ultimate Career Goal
- F. My Nursing Philosophy

II. Basic Nursing Education
Copy of work
Personal journal reflection

III. Continuing Nursing or Health-Related Education
Certificates of Completion
Program Brochures

IV. Licensure and Certification Documentation

V. Honors and Awards

VI. Professional Organization Activities

VII. Community Service Activities

The portfolio is a representation of a career over time. Updates can be done on an annual basis, so collect artifacts over time. Keep these in a safe place and organize them in folders with portfolio headings for careful selection later. Make sure to date all items added to the growing resource of information in order to verify the time frame in which to reference them. This will allow sequential placement of information in the portfolio. Use a mentor to help with review and critique of the portfolio. This individual should be experienced in the profession in order to give the best feedback. Don't take comments personally but work with the mentor to make the portfolio the best professional representation possible. Carefully review the document. This will allow you to look at your personal career in a reflective mode. Answer the following questions:

- Does the document accurately reflect my career to this point? If not, why not, and what can I do to change this representative document? (A mentor may be able to assist with this.)
- Am I where I want to be at this point in my career?
- What has contributed to my successes?
- What has not allowed me to progress to the degree I desire?
- What are some future activities that will promote continued growth toward identified goals?

Things to Include in the Portfolio

There are many ways to organize a portfolio. All generally start with a title page that includes your name, address, telephone number, e-mail address, program name, degree working to complete, and projected date of graduation or degree completion. A table of contents and introductory statement should follow this section. The introductory statement should include a one-page overview of the portfolio. Include dividers in order to allow for expansion of this document as progression is made from the educational arena to the professional one. Major components are identified in brief in Box 2. Specifics are identified in Box 3.

Specifically state goals succinctly, clearly, and directly (see Box 4 for examples). Describe goals in detail. Find a theme for this information. If the theme is to help people be specific in identifying which people (e.g., children, adults, the elderly). Expand on this theme to include which specific category (e.g., children with cancer, adult critical care patients, elderly in the community, etc.). Use specific personal experiences to illustrate the theme's evolution.

Box 3. Detailed Outline

I. Baseline Data
   A. Why I want to be a nurse (can begin by telling a personal statement that affected why you decided to
      pursue a career in nursing)
   B. People or experiences that inspired me to enter the profession
   C. Short-Term Goals (2–4 years) (present only professional goals)
   D. Long-Term Goals (5–10 years) (present only professional goals)
   E. Ultimate Career Goal (e.g., terminal degree desired, etc.)
   F. My Nursing Philosophy

II. Basic Nursing Education
   A. Copy of at least one paper or other project from each sophomore, junior, or senior year nursing course. If
      you have a pre-nursing component to your program of study, you can use a paper starting from a general
      studies course.
   B. A personal journal reflection of accomplishments at the end of each semester, such as: how have you
      changed, what was the most important thing you learned, what was your most interesting clinical
      experience?

III. Continuing Nursing or Health-Related Education (experiences beyond traditional course requirements, such
      as conferences and workshops, or self-directed independent study)
   A. Certificates of Completion
   B. Program Brochures: these should be for seminars or continuing education attended

IV. Licensure and Certification Documentation (e.g., start with CPR card, CNA certification, etc.)

V. Honors and Awards (include copies of letters of recommendation/commendation)

VI. Professional Organization Activities (include student organizations as well as other professional organizations)

VII. Community Service Activities (be sure to identify the name of the organization, city, and state of the
organization, purpose of the organization, and your role in the organization).

Information should be presented from a professional perspective in the portfolio. It is not appropriate to include personal goals such as getting married or moving to a specific part of the country. Goals should be well thought out and presented in a coherent manner that reflect precision and specifics. Arrange information in paragraph format that is a minimum of one paragraph (a minimum of one third of a page) which demonstrates thought and active reflection.

Organize information in an easy-to-read format that is grammatically correct. Guide the reader with all information included to the portfolio. Examples of academic papers should follow a specific form of writing such as the American Psychological Association (APA) or Modern Language Association (MLA) throughout. Use examples of the best work completed during pre-nursing and/or nursing courses.

The nursing philosophy statement should be developed carefully in a stepwise fashion (see Figure 3). The opening statement should introduce the reader to you as an individual. The ending statement needs to be a powerful conclusion to this philosophy. Make the final sentence memorable for the reader. The philosophy should reflect personal beliefs and justification for those beliefs.

Assemble all information in the portfolio in an easy-to-read format. Use a three-ring binder or specific portfolio purchased for this type of presentation. Type all dividers and all work in the portfolio. It may be possible to transition to an electronic portfolio, so keep information available in electronic format in a computer folder for later retrieval. This can also be subdivided using the same major headings as a three-ring binder. Don't forget to date all your information for accurate sequencing. This can be done by adding the date to the name of the saved file, which would allow you to eliminate altering any original work.

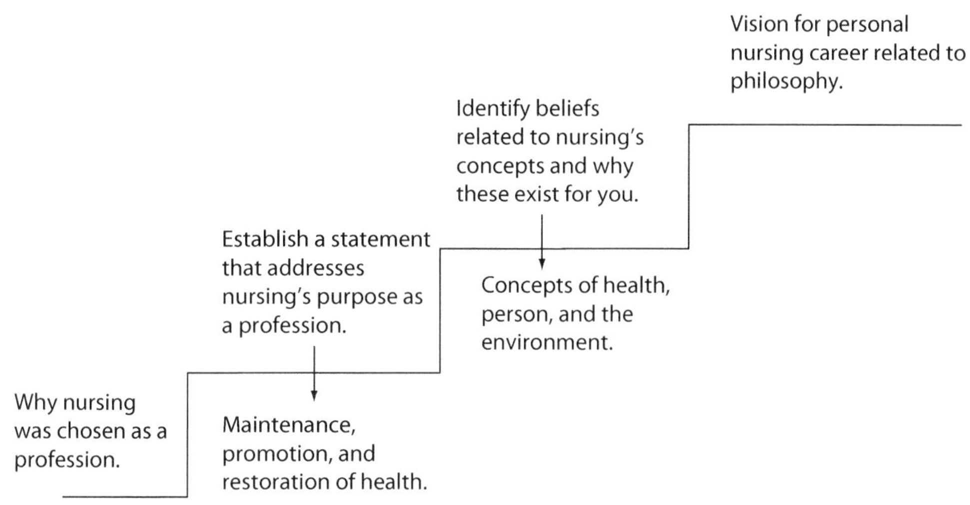

Figure 3. Steps to Developing a Nursing Philosophy

Proofread all information. Grammar and sentence structure are important to making a favorable impression. Structurally organize content to create a memorable impression. It is good to read information over a period of time in order to verify that all information has been included for a professional presentation with personal reflection and enthusiasm. Review and update the portfolio as personal and professional goals change over the years.

The First Job

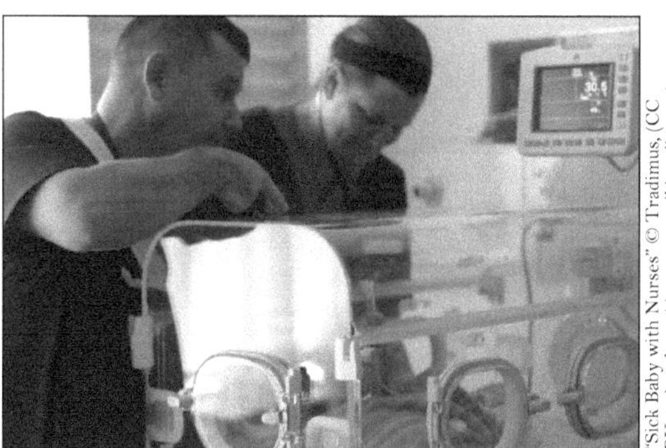

New graduates may look to facilities used for educational clinical sites as a potential first job. This has advantages for the organization and the nurse graduate. The organization has an opportunity to evaluate skills and potential for continued learning of the graduate nurse, and the graduate has the opportunity to evaluate compatibility with the organization's goals and philosophy.

Some organizations allow the new graduate to work within limitations on role responsibility and accountability. Salaries for these positions are often reduced, with salary and position increase upon verification of licensure. Following successfully obtaining licensure, the initials "RN" may be used to designate that registered nurse status has been achieved and approval granted by the state board of nursing. Patient care legal responsibility and accountability will also increase following licensure. This usually starts with an orientation to the organization and validation of skills to be used on the specific area of employment (acute or extended care). This begins annual events training, which many organizations require (e.g., fire management training, cardiopulmonary resuscitation training and certification, medication administration protocols, etc.). This orientation will include timed educational sessions that will educate the new nurse to computerized organizational components such as the electronic patient record, computerized medication administration system and laboratory/radiological data retrieval system. Orientation will include retrieval of computer access codes and log-ons, which should be kept confidential and not shared with anyone. These are unique to each nurse and may time stamp and electronically sign information entered into the system following log-on.

New employee orientation is usually performed in a classroom format. Information regarding care area specifics will usually be taught following new employment orientation. This is where new nurses enter the care area for orientation related to specialized equipment and skill that may be needed. At this time, the new RN may be paired with an experienced nurse to promote continued learning of area specifics. This time frame and peer collaboration situation is given different names by various organizations. It may be called preceptorship, mentorship, or nurse residency. The length of time for this orientation program can vary based on complexity and progression of the new graduate along the learning continuum. It may range from a few weeks to several months for more complex areas such as critical care or the emergency department.

This is an exciting time for the new RN. It is the culmination of years of study and work. It validates success and is just the beginning of a professional course of learning as health care continues to evolve.

Work Environments

What to Consider in a Work Environment

Work environments vary greatly from organization to organization based on type, structure, goals, and philosophical base. Choosing an environment that augments your personal philosophy is important. Many organizations have web-based information that gives the organization's history, organizational structure, philosophy, purpose, aim, departments for patient care delivery and employee information, among others. Take the time to go through this information available for review. Demonstration of some knowledge related to the organization demonstrates true interest in employment during an interview. It also allows you to identify questions that may need to be clarified prior to employment. For example, if you are interested in returning to school during the first two years of employment and you plan on working for this organization for a minimum of six years, identifying educational benefits would be important.

Salary is an important component to consider. Don't assume that salary is not negotiable. Of course, the more experience you have in an area of specialty the more bargaining power you have. The key is to do your homework. Take a look at posted salary ranges for the position of choice in the geographic and professional areas you are interested in for employment. Request the range and what components are considered when discussing this topic. Don't be shy. It is important to get this right the first time. Opportunities to discuss salary prior to beginning employment end when the contract is signed. Following acceptance of the contract, salary increases may only be based on strict identified components for the organization (e.g., obtaining certification in a specialty, cost-of-living raises, moving up to a new salary level on a structured position ladder, etc.).

Know yourself and what characteristics are important to personally augment in an organization for you to achieve professional satisfaction. You chose nursing because it fit certain personality traits. Preferences regarding a work environment can be just as important as choosing a career. Work to identify organizations that will allow you to continue and achieve identified career goals. Use the following form to help you with this (see Table 2).

Questions ranked #1 ____________________________
Questions ranked #2 ____________________________
Questions ranked #3 ____________________________

The Know-Your-Work-Preference Questionnaire can give you a start to identifying what you are looking for in an organization for employment and can facilitate looking in the right place for the right job. For example, if you completed the questionnaire as follows (see Table 3), you would look for a job in Atlanta, Georgia, because it would be close to family and friends. You would give preference to job openings in an organization that did surgeries but did not perform procedures that were against your religious convictions.

Just remember that it is important to work in an area that fulfills professional goals and personal needs. This will increase your success and enjoyment as a nurse.

Magnet Hospital Recognition Program Work Environments

One designation for excellence in organizations is the American Nurses Credentialing Center Magnet Recognition Program. This program grew out

Table 2. Know-Your-Work-Preference Questionnaire Instructions: Respond to the following items in the table.		
Questions	Rationale	Rank the Order of Importance Number (1, 2, or 3)
1. In what city and state would you like to work?	Why did you select these areas of the country?	
2. What type of organization do you want to work in?	Why did you select this type?	
3. Is distance from employer important?	Why?	
4. Are employment hours of work important?	Why?	
5. What hours would you prefer to work if the organization offers shift work for nurses? (e.g., two 12-hour shifts = 7 am–7 pm, or 7 pm–7 am; three– 8-hour shifts = 7 am–3 pm, 3 pm–11 pm, or 11 pm–7am, etc.)	Why did you select these hours?	
6. What specific area in the organization would you like to work?	Why this area?	
7. Do you have any convictions that would be a "deal breaker" when it comes to seeking employment?	What is the source of your convictions?	
8. Do you have any specific personality traits that are important to augment in your work area?	What are these?	

of a study to identify hospital work characteristics. The American Academy of Nursing (AAN) Task Force on Nursing Practice in Hospitals conducted this study in 1983 to identify work environments that were nursing and patient care focused. It looked to identify organizations that attracted, as well as retained, well-qualified nurses who promoted quality patient care. In this study, 163 hospitals participated, and of that number, 41 possessed qualities identified to have a greater capacity to attract and retain nurses. These hospitals were described as "magnet" hospitals.

Characteristics that distinguished these 41 hospitals from their counterparts are known as the "Forces of Magnetism." In 1990 the American Nurses Association (ANA) Board of Directors approved a proposal for the Magnet Hospital Recognition Program for Excellence in Nursing Services. This program was directly built on the 1983 study results that form the framework for the appraisal process.

Hospitals must meet all components in order to be considered for Magnet status. Following designation, the organization must maintain quality patient care, nursing excellence, and innovations in professional nursing practice in order to meet redesignation criteria. Characteristics of these facilities include a high number of nurses with bachelor/university degrees (41.8%56.72%). Many hospitals report longevity of

Table 3. Example of Completed Work Preference Questionnaire Instructions: Respond to the following items in the table.		
Questions	**Rationale**	**Rank the Order of Importance Number (1, 2, or 3)**
1. In what city and state would you like to work? ATLANTA, GA	CLOSE TO FAMILY & FRIENDS	1
2. What type of organization do you want to work in? HOSPITAL OR FREESTANDING SURGICENTER	WANT TO WORK IN SURGICAL AREA	1
3. Is distance from employer important? NO	HAVE OWN TRANSPORTATION	3
4. Are employment hours of work important? NO	SINGLE	3
5. What hours would you prefer to work if the organization offers shift work for nurses? (e.g., two 12-hour shifts = 7 am–7 pm, or 7 pm–7am; three– 8-hour shifts = 7 am–3pm, 3 pm–11 pm, or 11 pm–7am, etc.) DAYSHIFT	PREFER DAYTIME WORK	3
6. What specific area in the organization would you like to work? RECOVERY ROOM	LIKE TO WORK WITH PATIENTS AFTER SURGERY	3
7. Do you have any convictions that would be a "deal breaker" when it comes to seeking employment? YES	What is the source of your convictions? RELIGIOUS	1
8. Do you have any specific personality traits that are important to augment in your work area? YES	What are these?	2

nurses with an average employment range of 9.7 to 11 years. Turnover rates were low at 8.4% to 10.8%. Organizations that have achieved Magnet recognition are reported to have satisfied nurses who foster collaborative environments between nurses and among other health care members.

Summary

Nursing is a profession of tremendous possibilities and opportunities. Knowledge of initiatives and current care activities promotes safety for patient and provider. The profession uses a dynamic process of communication that allows the nurse to make a significant difference in the lives of the patients they care for. This unique profession is rewarding and allows growth and expansion of an individual personally

Table 4. Forces of Magnetism

Force	Explanation
1. Nursing Leadership Quality	Qualities include knowledge and risk-taking and vision for nursing service operational development. Leaders should exhibit advocacy and support for staff and patients. Bedside patient care should exhibit strong leadership qualities.
2. Structure of the Organization	Organizational structures are decentralized decision-making. This decision-making structure should be dynamic and responsive to necessary change for the best outcomes. There should be strong nursing representation evident in organizational structure. There is a system of shared decision making which involves nursing.
3. Style of Management	The health care organization supports participation which is also supported by nursing leadership. Engagement and feedback are encouraged at all levels within organizational staff. Individuals who hold nursing leadership positions are accessible and visible to promote communication. These leaders are committed to the promotion of effective communication.
4. Policies for Personnel and Programs	The organization exhibits competitive salaries and benefits. Staffing models demonstrate creativity and flexibility in an effort to support a safe environment that promotes physiological and psychological health. Staff policy development involves nursing personnel and support professional practice for nurses, balance of life and work and quality patient care delivery. Opportunities for professional growth exist within the organization.
5. Professional Care Models	Models of care promote nursing responsibility, accountability and autonomy in the coordination of direct patient care. Nurses are held accountable for their own practice. Care models provide for continuity while allowing for care across the patient continuum. These models address the provision of skilled nurses and resources needed to accomplish desired patient outcomes.
6. Quality of Care	Quality is a fundamental force for the organization and nursing within this organization. Nurses should hold leadership positions that will positively influence patient outcomes. Nurses perceive that they deliver high quality care to patients within the organization.
7. Quality Improvement	The organization is designed to provide for the measurement of quality outcomes. These outcomes allow for evaluation in order to improve patient care and services.
8. Organizational Consultation and Resources	There are adequate resources provided by the organization to support utilization of experts for consultation and management. These experts include those within the nursing field inclusive of advanced practice nurses. The organization encourages nurse involvement and peer interaction in professional organizations and community activities.
9. Nursing Autonomy	The nurse is expected to provide autonomous care that includes assessment and interventions based on professional competence, expertise and knowledge. Autonomous nursing care should be demonstrated through implementation of independent judgment consistent with professional nursing standards. Autonomous care should be delivered utilizing interdisciplinary and multidisciplinary approaches to patient care in all settings.
10. Community and Health Care Organizations	Partnerships should be developed that support improved patient outcomes. These strong partnerships should be collaborative and support healthy communities.
11. Academic Educational Support	Nurses should be involved in educational activities. Organizations should be open to various academic programs. Contractual agreements support this mutually beneficial relationship.
12. Nursing Image	Nurses should be viewed as integral members of the health care organization. Services they provide should be regarded as essential by other individuals on the health care team. Nurses should effectively influence processes that affect the entire organizational system.
13. Relationship Between Disciplines	Value should be placed on collaborative relationships within and among organizational disciplines. All members of the health care team should make essential and meaningful contributions to clinical outcome achievement which promotes mutual respect. Strategies to manage conflicts should be in place and effectively used then necessary

Force	Explanation
14. Professional Development	Staff personal and professional growth are valued and supported by the organization. Emphasis is placed on career development through formal education and professional certification. Clinical competency and leadership/management developed are promoted within the organization. Professional development programs have adequate human and fiscal resources.

Adapted from American Nurses Credentialing Center. www.nursecredentialing.org/Magnet/ProgramOverview/HistoryoftheMagnetProgram/ForcesofMagnetism.aspx.

and professionally. It is rewarding to hear yourself say the words "I am your nurse today."

References

Campbell, D., Cignetti, P., Melemyzer, B., Nettles, D., & Wyman, R. (2011). *How to Develop a Professional Portfolio: A Manual for Teachers.* Pearson: New Jersey.

National Council of State Boards of Nursing (NCSBN) (2006). Fast facts about alternate item formats and the NCLEX examination. Retrieved from https://www.ncsbn.org/01_08_04_Alt_Itm.pdf

Nursing Jobs. Nursing interview techniques. Retrieved from http://nursejobs.com/nursing-interview-questions.aspx

Priest, C. (2010). The benefits of developing a professional portfolio. Retrieved from http://www.naeyc.org/files/yc/file/201001/PriestWeb0110.pdf.

Scholastic. The professional portfolio. Retrieved from http://www2.scholastic.com/browse/article.jsp?id=4148

Chapter 14: Selected Nursing Career Options

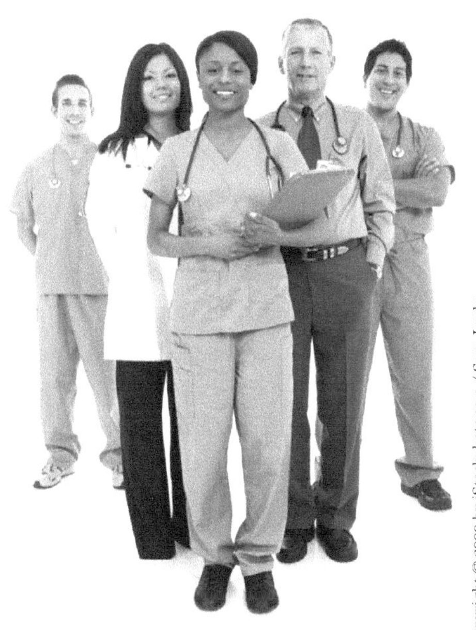

Nursing offers a variety of professional pathways. Upon completion of a nursing educational program, it is important to select an employment area of interest, one that you feel can promote the best process for socialization into the profession. Many new graduates start out in hospitals in an area of interest. As you progress through the years of educational preparation, it is important to identify areas that you find a match with—the ones that just feel right. This can give you a clue to areas that may be a good personal and professional complement. Organizations differ, and all career options are not available in all institutions. Some companies validate the expertise of individuals who apply for work through an agency. Some require satisfactory demonstration of knowledge, such as acquiring a specific score on a pharmacology test or an assessment that evaluates basic nursing care. As your experience and education increase, your career options increase significantly. This chapter will give you an introduction to some areas that are available to the new graduate nurse. It is not a complete listing of all potential areas in nursing.

Agency Nursing

Nurses who work in agencies register or sign up for a specific company that is usually outside of a health care organization. The company will designate areas of potential work based on experience. As an agency nurse, you may work in one of several health care organizations with which the company has a contractual agreement to supply nurses at times of shortage (e.g., employees on vacation, maternity leave, illness, etc.). As an agency employee you are paid directly by the company. It is important to familiarize yourself with policies and procedures for both the company and organization. If you travel to other parts of the country or the world, this is called Travel Nursing.

Critical Care Nursing

Critical nurses provide care for patients who are acutely and critically ill. Knowledge of advanced care management usually requires extended orientation times for organizations who hire new graduates into this area. Orientation may be from six months to one year in order to build knowledge and confidence to manage patients experiencing life-threatening situations (e.g., cardiac or respiratory arrest). More specific areas in critical care include those specifically devoted to care of cardiac patients (Coronary Care Unit–CCU) , surgical patients (Surgical Intensive Care Unit–SICU), neurological patients (Neurological Intensive Care Unit–NICU), etc. Additional information can be obtained from the American Association of Critical Care Nurses (AACN) at http://www.aacn.org/.

Emergency Department

Nurses who work in the emergency department see patients who present for various complications, from minor complications to life-threatening ones. These nurses must be able to quickly assess patients, provide independent and interdependent interventions, and evaluate patient outcomes. Nurses work with patients and families as they experience illness, injury, and crisis. This area can be a high-intensity area in which to work. Some emergency departments manage trauma patients who arrive in critical condition by helicopter and require intense lifesaving measures. Additional information can be obtained from the Emergency Nurses Association (ENA) at http://www.ena.org.

Flight Nursing

A flight nurse is a registered nurse with intensive/critical care nursing experience as well as emergency nursing. This type of care manages patients with a variety of emergencies under some very difficult situations. Transport may require initial treatment in remote areas under treacherous conditions in various parts of the country. Collaborative patient management may include teams of nurses and physicians while in flight as well as ground health care members. Flight nurses respond to transport critically injured individuals by helicopter or plane to trauma centers. These critical patients are aggressively managed during transport. Flight nurses are key members of medical disaster teams. Additional information can be obtained from the Air and Service Transport Nurses Association (ASTNA) at http://www.astna.org/.

Geriatric Nursing

Geriatric nurses care for elderly patients in a number of settings, which include the patient's home, extended care facilities, and hospitals. Geriatric nurses work to improve overall health and quality of life for older individuals while working to maintain independent care. They work directly with patients who are experiencing health concerns that are age related. Many older patients have multiple complex disease processes that pose a challenge to this type of nursing care. Patient education and management of care are essential to this population. The geriatric nurse is committed to providing high-quality, culturally sensitive care. Additional information can be obtained from the American Geriatrics Society (AGS) at http://www.americangeriatrics.org/.

Home Health Nursing

Home health nurses provide intermittent care services to patients at home. These nurses travel to urban and rural sites to give care to individuals who do not require institutional care on a constant basis. They work with individuals who are being managed at home from illness, accident, or childbirth. These may be individuals who are restricted to their homes and cannot travel for care. The home health nurse works collaboratively with other care providers and may directly supervise assistants. Additional information can be obtained from the Home Health Nurses Association (HHNA) at http://www.hhna.org/.

Military Nursing

Military nurses work in a variety of settings, ranging from family practice at a homeland military base to providing emergency care for the wounded in the field during time of war. All services currently have a branch that includes nurses. These branches are called corps. A corps is a military command whose members share a common mission and are grouped together. These nurses serve in the military and hold military rank. Military nurses serve in the Army, Navy, Air Force, and Coast Guard. Additional information can be obtained about the Army Nurse Corps from http://www.goarmy.com/cl2.html, about the Navy Nurse Corps Association from http://www.nnca.org/, about the Air Force Nurse Corps from http://www.airforce.

com/ - select careers, and the Coast Guard from http://www.gocoastguard.com/ will need to contact an office for specific information regarding nursing.

Neonatal Nursing

Neonatal nurses provide care for newborn infants up to 28 days old while supporting the family. They must have astute assessment skills and knowledge of the care required for infants. Some organizations assess nursing skill abilities, pharmacological skills which include medication calculation, knowledge of intravenous lines, and cardiopulmonary resuscitation in the newborn population following an extensive orientation period. Neonatal nurses critically assess the patient to ensure good health, provide preventive care to prevent illness, and care for ill infants. The neonatal nurse is responsible for anticipating, preventing, diagnosing, and minimizing illness in newborns. There are various levels of the nurseries that neonatal nurses may work in. These include: Level I = healthy newborn nursery, Level II = intermediate care or special care nursery, or Level III – neonatal intensive care. Additional information can be obtained from the National Association of Neonatal Nurses (NANN) at http://www.nann.org/.

Occupational Health Nursing

The occupational health nurse is also called an employee health nurse and health promotion nurse among other names that may be specific to an organization. This type of nurse is responsible for maintaining the health and wellness of employees in an organization. They focus on health, safety, and productivity of employees. They not only treat illnesses that affect employee productivity, but are often responsible for maintaining wellness programs and activities for a business. Depending on the employer, an occupational health nurse may provide emergency care, prepare accident reports, and arrange for further care if necessary. They can offer health counseling, assist with health examinations and immunizations, and assess work environments to identify potential health or safety problems. The occupational health nurse is responsible for improving, protecting, maintaining, and restoring the health of employees. By providing this care for employees, the occupational health nurse is able to influence the health of the business. Additional information can be obtained from the American Association of Occupational Nurses, Inc. (AAOHN) at https://www.aaohn.org/.

Office Nursing

An office nurse may also be called a medical assistant. The office nurse is responsible for assisting in the delivery of health care and patient care management based on the specific office specialty which is governed by the physician or nurse practitioner. This includes retrieval of historical information which can assist in physician management. Office nurses obtain vital signs and other laboratory or demographic patient information (e.g., height, weight, etc.). They can assist in the preparation of patients for examination and delivery of care. They also assist in delivery of care, which can include minor surgical procedures, if these are part of the practice.

Oncology Nursing

Oncology nurses provide health care for cancer patients of all ages and during all stages of treatment from diagnosis to remission or death. The spectrum of care this nurse provides includes direct care delivery to education of patients and families. The oncology nurse also works to coordinate care between the many health care team members that may be necessary to promote quality of life for the oncology patient. They work to develop realistic goals and objectives for patient outcomes and are usually very involved in patient education to assist with management of the side effects of interventions for the patient's specific type of cancer treatment. Additional information can be obtained from the Oncology Nursing Society (ONS) at http://www.ons.org/.

Pediatric Nursing

Pediatric nurses care for infants, children, and adolescents in all aspects of health care. This care is specialized because this is a unique population with different needs. Pediatric nurses must deal with growth and development as well as illness and injury. They must be skilled at communicating and working with children to reduce confusion and fear. They work with families as well as infants, children, and adolescents. They also serve as educators to families in an effort to promote wellness in children. Pediatric nurses practice in a variety of settings, including hospitals, clinics, schools, and the home. Additional information can be obtained from the Society of Pediatric Nurses (SPN) at http://www.pedsnurses.org/.

Perioperative Nursing

Perioperative nurses work in preoperative, intraoperative, and postoperative areas in tertiary care hospitals, community and rural hospitals, day surgery units, and specialized clinics with a multidisciplinary team of health care providers. They often provide total care in preoperative and postoperative areas. Perioperative nurses may have specialized positions in the operative suite and serve as a scrub nurse or individual who is dressed to handle sterile instruments and supplies and pass them to the surgeon during the actual procedure, or a circulating nurse who serves to manage the overall care and helps maintain a safe, comfortable patient environment. Preoperative functions of the perioperative nurse are aimed at preparing the patient for a surgical procedure, and postoperative functions deal with patient care following the procedure. This is the recovery phase of care to discharge to a specific care area or home. Additional information can be obtained from the Association of periOperative Registered Nurses (AORN) at http://www.aorn.org/.

Psychiatric Nursing

Psychiatric nurses serve as integral members of a mental health interdisciplinary team for patient management. They provide care for patients and families with acute or chronic psychiatric and mental illnesses. This complex type of care requires the nurse to administer medications, monitor treatment interventions, and be an active participant in the patient's treatment plan. These nurses practice in a variety of settings, such as hospitals and institutions. Additional information can be obtained from the International Society of Psychiatric-Mental Health Nurses (ISPN) at http://www.ispn-psych.org/.

Public Health Nursing

Public health nurses provide comprehensive nursing services in preventive health, home health, and clinic programs to individuals, families, and communities. They travel to patient homes in urban and rural settings to collect referral information and conduct home visits to determine client needs. They develop individualized plans of care based on needs assessment and manage and coordinate community services to provide a multidisciplinary approach to resolution of needs. They work with individuals, families, and communities to find viable, accessible solutions to community health concerns. They work with local resources, expressing community health concerns to local health planners and policy makers, and assist members of the community to voice their own problems and concerns. Additional information can be obtained from the American Public Health Association (APHA)–Nursing at http://www.apha.org/membergroups/sections/aphasections/phn/.

School Nursing

School nurses work with students and school faculty, providing health care and other support in an in-school environment. The work setting extends from elementary school to university level education. School nurses manage all student and faculty situations, which include monitoring the environment for diseases, administration of medications, assessment and intervention for illnesses and injuries, collaborating with other health professionals to promote the health and educational success of students, and providing leadership and education in promoting nursing as a profession in the school environment. Additional information can be obtained from the National Association of School Nurses (NASN) at http://www.nasn.org/.

Travel Nursing

A travel nurse works for an agency and takes travel assignments inside or outside of the United States. In this country, they can work in local hospitals on a shift assignment or in hospitals across the country for approximately three months. These time periods can vary greatly. They work in hospitals that are usually experiencing an extreme nursing shortage, and working conditions can vary greatly from one assignment to the next. These nurses are usually highly paid and enjoy generous benefits, which can include sign-on bonuses and paid housing while on assignment, since their services are in high demand. They may work in any specialty area for which they are qualified, which can encompass the emergency department, critical care unit, postoperative care unit, surgical area, or almost any other nursing specialty. Additional information can be obtained from the American Travel Health Nurses Association (ATHNA) at http://www.athna.org/.

Transplant Nursing

Transplant nurses work in a variety of settings, and function in one of the two main areas of transplant: procurement and clinical. Procurement involves actually retrieving the organ. This nurse would work with an organ procurement agency and be a member of an interdisciplinary team. These nurses usually have a background in critical care. The nurses work to optimize harvesting (retrieval) of various organs, functioning as a liaison to promote the best results for retrieval and delivery to the patient waiting to receive the organ. Various body parts that may be retrieved for transplant include, but are not limited to: liver, kidney, pancreas, corneas, heart, and lungs. Clinical positions may be nurses with skill and managerial experience. This area of transplant requires the individual to have good problem-solving skills, be detail oriented, able to multitask effectively, be self-motivated, and have excellent verbal and written communications skills due to the intense emotional nature of the job. Additional information can be obtained from the International Transplant Nurses Society (ITNS) at http://www.itns.org/.

Trauma Nursing

Trauma nurses care for patients in emergency departments or critical care settings experiencing the results of a life-threatening traumatic situation. These nurses generally care for patients who have suffered severe trauma, such as motor vehicle accidents, gunshot wounds, stabbings, assaults, or other traumatic injuries. This area of nursing is high intensity and requires immediate assessment, intervention, and evaluation on a continuous basis. Patient stabilization is an interdisciplinary effort. These nurses need good communication skills to deal with family members during this highly emotionally charged time. Additional information can be obtained from the Society of Trauma Nurses (STN) at http://www.traumanurses.org/.

Urology Nursing

Urology nurses provide guidance and treatment for all individuals across the lifespan in the specialty of urology (deals with the urinary system). They work in a variety of settings from offices to clinics, retrieving patient historical information, performing examinations, interpreting diagnostic studies, and managing bladder diseases that cause dysfunction and incontinence. These can include cancer, infertility, incontinence, plastic surgery, urological repair, etc. Urology nurses are also focused on patient education so they need good communication skills, since this system can be personal and intimate to individuals. Additional information can be obtained from the American Nephrology Nurses' Association (ANNA) at http://www.annanurse.org and the Society of Urologic Nurses and Associates (SUNA) at http://www.suna.org.

Women's Health

Women's health nurses work to facilitate health promotion and disease prevention of women in various health care settings. These nurses work with women in all stages of life and must adjust to incorporate family and community, since these issues affect women emotionally and psychologically. Women's health nurses work with women in obstetrics, gynecology, with health promotion activities (e.g., mammograms, pap smears, etc.), with reproductive health, and other general health issues that affect women. Nurses work to initiate gender focused assessments and interventions. Patient education and follow-up are key components in this type of nursing. Additional information can be obtained from the Association of Women's Health, Obstetric and Neonatal Nurses (AWHONN) at http://www.awhonn.org/awhonn /.

Nursing Career Options That Require Advanced Practice Status or Additional Education

An advanced practice nurse has a minimum of a master's degree in nursing. These career options are marked with an asterisk* for ease of identification. Other careers require additional continuing educational programs.

Anesthesia—Certified Registered Nurse Anesthetist (CRNA)*

A certified registered nurse anesthetist is an advanced practice nurse who specializes in anesthesia care for individuals of all ages. They collaborate with anesthesiologists, surgeons, and other health care professionals to deliver anesthesia for medical and surgical procedures in hospital, clinic, and office settings. They can work in specific areas, such as hospital or outpatient surgical operating rooms, labor and delivery units, critical care units, and various physician specialty offices (e.g., plastic surgeons, dentists, ophthalmologists, pain management, etc.). They manage anesthesia needs during all phases of patient interaction. They interact with patients and families in the delivery of care. Additional information can be obtained from the American Association of Nurse Anesthetists (AANA) at http://www.aana.com/.

Clinical Nurse Specialists*

The clinical specialist uses case management as a collaborative interdisciplinary process for patient care. Clinical nurse specialists can work in several roles that can include clinical practice, consulting, management, teaching, or research. They are skilled at using assessment, planning, facilitation, and advocacy for exercising options and services to meet individual health needs in inpatient and outpatient settings. These individually designed health care programs efficiently use available resources to promote quality cost-effective outcomes. Additional information can be obtained from the National Association of Clinical Nurse Specialists (NACNS) at http://www.nacns.org/.

Instructor/Professor*—Schools/Colleges of Nursing

The nursing instructor has advanced education in a specialty area. These individuals are either master's degree or doctorally prepared and teach in areas of nursing based on their earned degree. These areas can include any course in a nursing program that is didactic (classroom) or clinically based. Academic programs usually require that in order to teach, the nurse must have a degree one level higher than the level for which they teach (e.g., individuals teaching in a baccalaureate program must have a minimum of a master's degree, and individuals teaching in a master's program must have a minimum of a doctorate). Faculty must remain current in order to teach appropriate, relevant information that will assist the new graduate to NCLEX-RN success and effective transitioning to a new job. There is no specific organization for nursing faculty, but the organization that promotes higher nursing education is the American Association of Colleges of Nursing (AACN) and can be located at http://www.aacn.nche.edu/.

Forensic Nursing

Forensic nurses specialize in providing care for victims and perpetrators of crime. They collect evidence after crimes occur and provide medical care to patients within the prison system. They are an integral part of the legal system and provide consultation to both medical and legal organizations. They work on cases that can include suspected child abuse, elder abuse, or sexual assault. Forensic nurses help law enforcement build cases against suspected criminals and serve as expert witnesses in court trials. Additional information can be obtained from the International Association of Forensic Nurses (IAFN) at http://www.iafn.org/

Holistic Nursing

Holistic nurses engage in providing care that addresses all areas of care and incorporates traditional and alternative medicine (e.g., massage, music therapy, acupressure, therapeutic touch, guided imagery, relaxation, etc.). Holistic nursing focuses on the principle that the whole person must be considered in order to effectively treat an individual. This includes physiological, psychological, and sociological factors. The holistic nurse provides care that incorporates the patient's health beliefs and values. They integrate self-care, spirituality, and reflection into their daily nursing care activities to promote wellness that incorporates the whole person (body, mind, and spirit). Additional information can be obtained from the American Holistic Nurses Association (AHNA) at http://www.ahna.org/.

Informatics Nursing*

Informatics nursing combines nursing with information technology. They manage data repositories that may contain confidential patient information. They promote information retrieval from the organization to the end-user to assist in the delivery of patient care. The informatics nurse works closely with users of clinical information systems within an organization. They serve a key role in planning initiatives that relate to nurse-based systems or other software or hardware components that interface with these systems. They evaluate clinical information systems from the user's perspective in order to manage workflow in collaboration with organizational project managers and directors. They work to verify that information systems are clinically applicable and consistent with professional nursing standards. Additional information can be obtained from the American Nursing Informatics Association (ANIA) at http://www.ania-caring.org/.

Legal Nursing

Legal nursing combines law and nursing. Attorneys rarely have knowledge of medical terminology and when dealing with medical malpractice and personal injury cases, they require assistance in reviewing patient chart information. They assist with translating medical records, validating the significance and appropriateness of nursing interventions, and other health care issues. Many legal nurses have several years of experience and advanced degrees (master's degree or doctorate), which adds credibility to their testimony as expert witnesses regarding the standards and guidelines for care. They assist with identifying strategies for resolutions in health care cases, educate attorneys in differentiating key facts from just general information, interview witnesses, draft legal documents, and provide support during legal proceedings. Additional information can be obtained from the American Association of Legal Nurse Consultants (AALNC) at http://www.aalnc.org/

Nurse Midwives*

Nurse midwives have an advanced degree that has prepared them to deal specifically with childbirth and prenatal and postpartum care. They manage the physical, emotional, and mental state of the mother throughout the birthing process and work to reduce the use of adjunction devices or medications. Nurse midwives work with women throughout labor and delivery. They deal with the natural birthing process only and are not qualified to perform a cesarean section, should it be required. Following delivery, they perform postpartum examinations to validate the health status of mother and baby. They may work in a clinic, alone, or as a member of a group of nurse midwives in collaboration with a physician. They perform postpartum visits and educate the mother to promote ongoing health. Additional information can be obtained from the American College of Nurse Midwives (ACNM) at http://www.midwife.org/.

Nurse Practitioner*

A nurse practitioner is an advanced practice nurse who has completed education at the masters or doctoral level. They can deliver primary care delivery for individuals throughout the lifespan. They can diagnose, treat (including prescribing medications), consult, provide follow-up, and referral for a variety of disease processes. Some can perform limited procedures, such as suturing open wounds. They educate patients and families about preventive care and treatments. They may work in clinics, offices or a hospital, in some states. They may also work independently or interdependently. They can participate in the care of inpatient and outpatients. They are responsible for patient record accuracy and managing records according to standards and policies. There are many different types of nurse practitioners: Family, Pediatric, Adult, Geriatric, Women's Health Care, Neonatal, Acute Care, and Occupational Health. Additional information can be obtained from the American Academy of Nurse Practitioners (AANP) at http://www.aanp.org/AANPCMS2 or the American College of Nurse Practitioners (ACNP) at http://www.acnpweb.org.

Research Nursing

Research nurses work in hospitals or other companies with strong research initiatives (e.g., pharmaceutical companies, medical technology companies). They perform both clinical and basic research to develop a research- or evidence-based approach to patient management. They need a good background in assessment and patient management in order to make changes to the plan of care based on the patient responses and stabilize patient parameters that may result from side effects of the research intervention. They develop plans of care and treatment protocols that incorporate components of the research process and monitor patient responses to interventions. They work with individuals across the lifespan and with all types of illnesses in an effort to promote quality of life. Their research can focus on pain management, reduction of risks for disease and disability, and promotion of a healthy lifestyle in individuals with chronic diseases. Additional information can be obtained from the Western Institute of Nursing Research (WIN) at http://www.winursing.org/, the Midwest Nursing Research Society (MNRS) at http://www.mnrs.org/, the Southern Nursing Research Society (SNRS) at http://snrs.org, and the Eastern Nursing Research Society (ENRS) at http://www.enrs-go.org/.

Summary

Nursing is a career of immense challenges and joys. It requires continued learning and effort to give the highest level of nursing care to individuals, families, and communities. Regardless of the type of nursing you decide, it will give you years of personal and professional satisfaction.

References

American Academy of Nurse Practitioners at http://www.aanp.org/AANPCMS2

American College of Nurse Practitioners at http://www.acnpweb.org

Air and Service Transport Nurses Association at http://www.astna.org/

Air Force Nurse Corps from http://www.airforce.com/

American Association of Colleges of Nursing at http://www.aacn.nche.edu/

American Association of Critical Care Nurses at http://www.aacn.org/.

American Association of Legal Nurse Consultants at http://www.aalnc.org/

American Association of Nurse Anesthetists at http://www.aana.com/

American Association of Occupational Nurses, Inc. at https://www.aaohn.org/

American College of Nurse Midwives at http://www.midwife.org/

American Nephrology Nurses' Association http://www.annanurse.org

Association of periOperative Registered Nurses at http://www.aorn.org/

American Public Health Association—Nursing at http://www.apha.org/membergroups/sections/aphasections/phn/

American Geriatrics Society at http://www.americangeriatrics.org/.

American Holistic Nurses Association at http://www.ahna.org/

American Nursing Informatics Association at http://www.ania-caring.org/

American Travel Health Nurses Association at http://www.athna.org/

Army Nurse Corps from http://www.goarmy.com/cl2.html

Association of Women's Health, Obstetric and Neonatal Nurses at http://www.awhonn.org/awhonn/

Coast Guard from http://www.gocoastguard.com/

Eastern Nursing Research Society at http://www.enrs-go.org/

Emergency Nurses Association at http://www.ena.org.

Home Health Nurses Association at http://www.hhna.org/.

International Association of Forensic Nurses at http://www.iafn.org/

International Society of Psychiatric-Mental Health Nurses at http://www.ispn-psych.org/

International Transplant Nurses Society at http://www.itns.org/

Midwest Nursing Research Society at http://www.mnrs.org/

Navy Nurse Corps Association from http://www.nnca.org/

National Association of Clinical Nurse Specialists at http://www.nacns.org/

National Association of Neonatal Nurses at http://www.nann.org/

National Association of School Nurses at http://www.nasn.org/

Oncology Nursing Society at http://www.ons.org/

Society of Pediatric Nurses at http://www.pedsnurses.org/

Society of Trauma Nurses at http://www.traumanurses.org/

Society of Urologic Nurses and Associates at http://www.suna.org

Southern Nursing Research Society at http://snrs.org

Western Institute of Nursing Research at http://www.winursing.org/

Chapter 15: Nursing's Future

The Road Ahead

I t is difficult to envision what nursing will evolve to encompass from its past but it will surely be an exciting and forward-moving profession. Nursing's professionalization has certainly found its niche in evidence-based patient management, and it continues to move in this direction. Nurse researchers have evolved and continue to develop foundational theoretical perspectives that give recognition to the science of nursing. They continue to study concepts related to the phenomenon of concern to nursing from a quantitative and qualitative perspective. These include research of numbers that relate to care (quantitative research) as well as attitudes which are holistic in nature (qualitative research). Results of this type of research ensure that the nursing profession will have a scientific base for care compassion and competence in patient management.

The Impact of Health Care's Future Impact on Nursing

Significant changes have occurred in the United States that impact the future of health care and nursing management. These trends evolve around (a) management of health care costs; (b) access to care for all individuals; (c) genomics and nanotechnology; (d) and cultural changes in the patient population. The following paragraphs will give more detail about each trend and its impact on nursing.

Health Care Costs and Access to Care

Changes to the health care system are constantly being made by local, state, and federal government agencies in an effort to increase access to care. The United States continues to allocate numerous resources to care. Health care costs have continued an uphill climb (see Figure 1).

In 2010 health care costs surpassed $2.6 trillion, more than a tenfold increase since 1980 and more than three times the 1990 costs of $714 billion (Centers for Medicare and Medicaid Services, 2010). This year also saw per-resident costs of approximately $7,681, which represented 16.2% of the nation's Gross Domestic Product (GDP).

Without reform, these costs are anticipated to continue to rise. The 2010 federal plan initiated by President Obama to implement care for all Americans has been met with varying degrees of acceptance. This plan is stated to promote affordable health

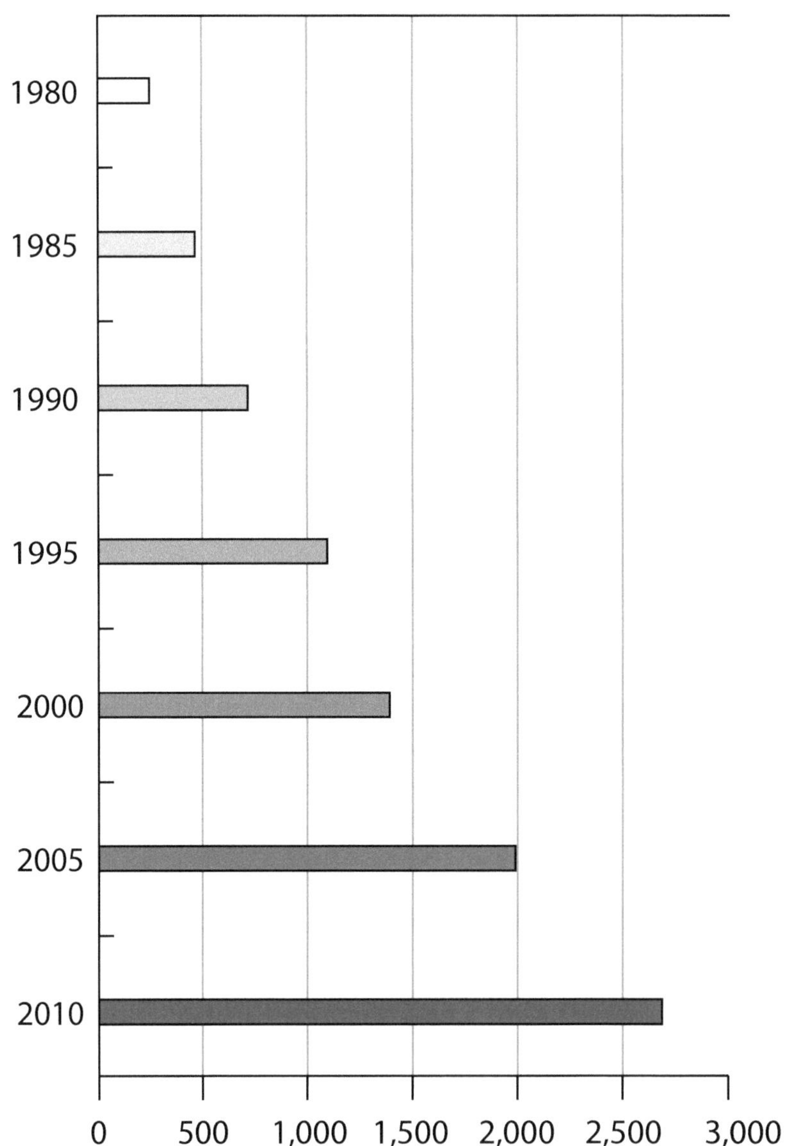

Figure 1. United States Health Care Expenditures from 1980–2010

care, accountability of insurers, expansion of coverage to all individuals, and sustain the health care system over time. This plan proposes to reduce deductibles for preventive services that will increase access at a foundational level and allow for patient education, a foundational component of nursing care. There are many pro and con perspectives on this care. The only certainty of this plan is that it will change the face of health care for all.

States have begun to implement changes due to the Affordable Care Act. This act increased the number of children with health care. It also worked to eliminate health care limits, both annual and lifetime, for individuals. This change allowed young adults to remain on their parents; health insurance up to and including the age of 25. This act also improved access to preventive services recommended for maintenance of health and well-being. This act also included beneficial changes for senior Americans, allowing them to access medications at 50% discounts. This one act alone would reduce the outlay of pharmaceutical monies for a section of the population who live on a fixed income and often have numerous conditions that require medicinal intervention.

In the current health care system, no one can be turned away from emergency departments if they present with a medical emergency. As a result, due to the cost of preventive care, the uninsured are more often treated in emergency rooms. This number for the uninsured is significantly higher than insured individuals. Many uninsured do not have access to treatment for conditions when they first occur, so they elect to wait until situations exist that require intervention. At this time, their health care situation requires more urgent intervention and the cost of care is significantly higher. The expense of emergency room care   Emergency room care is very expensive—it would cost less to either pay for preventive health care or treat the health problem before it became a more serious situation.

Nurses will have challenges to care based on alterations in care that promote early discharge by Health Maintenance Organizations (HMOs) and Preferred Provider Organizations (PPOs). Some are also promoting care activities that prompt individuals to self-manage diseases such as hypertension (high blood pressure) and diabetes. These encourage dietary as well as medication compliance in order to prevent innovations needed to manage complications such as heart disease and poor circulation.

Nurses will have increased patient care responsibilities inclusive of preventive patient education in order to promote self-management and reduced interventional care after disease. This follows the Healthy People 2020 initiative to provide scientifically based national objectives to promote health and prevent disease. National health care objective strategies are just a few mechanisms that have been, and will continue to be, used as part of the techniques nurses will use to gauge health care. These will allow nurses to develop theoretical perspectives that advance a model of care that promotes a proactive primary health care focus. This will concentrate on prevention rather than as a reaction to acute care issues. Nurses will be influential in shaping this type of health care system through research and theory development of key concepts. This will serve to validate nursing's professional importance to cost containment through validation of the best mechanism of care.

Genomics and Nanotechnology
Genomics

Genomics focuses on structure of the genome. This focal point moves toward identification and mapping of genes and sequencing DNA in organisms. Genomics also focuses on interactions of genes with each other and the environment. It has become an important part of diagnosis, prognosis, risk management, and treatment of clinical conditions in humans. Genomics is identified as a factor in the Ten Leading Causes of Death in 2007.

1. Heart disease
2. Cancer
3. Stroke (cerebrovascular diseases)
4. Chronic lower respiratory diseases
5. Accidents (unintentional injuries)
6. Alzheimer's disease
7. Diabetes
8. Influenza and pneumonia
9. Nephritis, nephrotic syndrome, and nephrosis
10. Septicemia

From http://www.cdc.gov/nchs/fastats/deaths.htm

This study of the relationship between genes, the environment, and individual behaviors allow researchers to identify why some individuals develop certain illnesses while others do not when exposed to the same factors. Family health history information can also help identify individuals who may be at higher risk of certain illnesses. A better understanding of genetic composition and family history can help health care providers identify, develop, and evaluate interventions that can improve individual health and prevent illness. Nurses will have a significant role in genomics, as retrieval of historical information has always been part of a foundation of nursing care. Nurse researchers and clinicians will work collaboratively in order to address issues that emerge as a result of genetic evaluation and testing. Working through the nursing process, nurses will improve health through implementation of genomics as a foundation for care.

Nanotechnology

Nanotechnology is just one technological innovation that will continue to advance health care. It will be very beneficial in diagnosis, prevention, and treatment of disease

Table 1.

Nursing Process	Genomic Activity
Assessment	Historical retrieval of detailed personal information and family history.
	Historical data targeted to information specific to an illness that patient presented for intervention.
	Family pedigree information obtained to outline and highlight inheritance patterns, which assist in detailed patient assessment.
Planning	Collaborative construction of individualized treatment plans inclusive of patient education.
Intervention	Collaborative intervention mechanisms initiated with physicians, genetic counselors, and other care providers based on individualized treatment plans.
Evaluation	Determination of the degree to which education, care, and support have been successfully implemented and to what degree these activities have addressed intervention for the identified problem(s).

processes. This technology will provide individual identification of disease before it is apparent in the body. This will allow health care to provide care from a preventable direction instead of reactive treatment following disease diagnosis and a subsequent struggle for management. Diagnosing in nanotechnology will provide effective monitoring of potential disease processes rather than treating these diseases after they have occurred and caused irreparable damage to body organs. Identifying the genetic makeup of the patient will allow health care providers the ability to prescribe and manage personalized preventive interventions. Patient treatments now entail the use of standard procedures and are not genetically patient based. Nanotechnology can provide individualized treatment plans that include specific medication doses that are truly unique for the person, and not within a designated range. A greater understanding of the genetics behind disease and response to treatment can allow for tailored health care treatments. Nanotechnology can lead to earlier diagnosis, which can result in more successful outcomes. Advances in bioassays (procedures for determining the biological activity of a substance) offer the potential to identify disease-causing microbes long before an individual presents symptoms of illness. Advanced monitoring can identify if treatment has been successful or if further alternate treatments are necessary. This can lead to improved quality of life and add to cost-effective interventions, which could reduce the overall cost of individualized health care.

Cultural Changes in the Patient Population

Culture is defined as a system which builds a social group. This system consists of attitudes, beliefs and behaviors that are shared, learned and passed on over generations. The resulting social group develops specific perceptions and responses that influence world perceptions and decision-making. It affects how people perceive the world around them. All individuals have a culture which influences how they think and feel. Culture also affects how they respond to illness and interact with caregivers.

The U. S. is a tossed salad of different cultures in that each culture retains their individual characteristics and harmoniously reside together. Cultures vary from state to state and can even change considerably from neighborhood to neighborhood.

According to the U.S Census Bureau, in 2009 the U.S. had 39 million foreign-born residents which represented a rate three times higher than Russia which ranks second in the list but lower than Australia and Canada. In 2010, of the 310 million residents in the U.S., two-thirds were non-Hispanic white and 20% were Hispanic or Asian. With continuation of the current trend in cultural changes, by 2050 the percent of non-Hispanic whites will decline to approximately 52% from 66%, Blacks will remain constant at 13% and Hispanics will increase to 29% from 16%.

Various cultures bring with them different practices and beliefs about healthcare. It is important for the nurse to learn and be aware of cultural differences. Since people are different, even among cultures traditional differences may exist. Since cultures can be clustered in various segments of the U.S. the nurse should be familiar with those specific cultures within their work domain. It is important for the nursing careplan to address patient cultural perspectives. The following list will give you some idea about culture and healthcare.

- Age—The perspective of age and culture are intertwined. Many cultures see geriatric individuals as persons who have increased in wisdom. The number of aging persons is increasing in many cultures (centurion boomer generation). These people may also have very traditional perspectives of health care, viewing physicians as guardians of their care and unquestionably follow directions. This may result in individuals failing to notify health care providers of adverse effects of medications or interventions. Patient education should be carefully validated emphasizing patient understanding by having them restate information.
- Alternative Medicine—The degree of allopathic medicine use and the use of alternative medicine will greatly vary by culture and individuals within cultures. Alternative medicine may include, but are not limited to, the use of acupuncture, aromatherapy, Chinese medicine, diet and nutrition, guided imagery, herbal therapies, homeopathy, and home remedies. Many people recognize the mind/body connection. It is important to respect thought processes and alternative medicine techniques that the patient feels will facilitate their wellness. Working to blend these two health care techniques may be a challenge.
- Culture Risk and Diseases—Specific disease risk patterns have been correlated to cultural practices. Black women suffer disproportionately when it comes to cardiovascular disease, stroke and premature death. Although heart disease and stroke are leading causes of death in Whites, Blacks, Asian, Hispanic and Native Americans, Blacks and Mexican American women are more likely to have risk factors than White women. Diabetes is more common among Blacks and Hispanics. High cholesterol does not follow this pattern. In general White women are more likely to be diagnosed with high cholesterol. Being familiar with cultural disease risk patterns should be taken into consideration and used when developing patient education.

- Diet—Culture will dictate the type of foods that are acceptable to consume. Palates are determined in part by customary foods consumed. One food may be acceptable in one culture but not included in the usual food eaten by another (e.g., Kimchi which is a traditional Korean super-spicy fermented dish of vegetables). It is important to set realistic dietary goals by considering traditional cultural foods.
- Eye Contact—Some cultures may see avoiding eye contact as a sign of respect, a way to avoid inappropriate eye contact of the opposite gender or prevent invasion of another individual's personal space. This should not be interpreted as lack of interest in the care activity or an act of aggression.
- Personal Space—Even among traditional Westerners this space can vary but is typically thought to be approximately 24 inches surrounding a person. This space is very specific for many cultures and invasion of this space can be viewed as an intrusion which can affect nurse-patient interaction.
- Touch—Some cultures stress modesty and touching body parts that are normally clothed is very uncomfortable. Touching the head may even be seen as a sign of disrespect. Touching among family members (including hugging or holding hands) may be welcomed while touching between strangers may be prohibited. Professional touching should be purposeful and firm.

It is important for the nurse to understand the link between culture and health. This link is critical to the development of care delivery and an effective patient outcome.

Clinical Wisdom

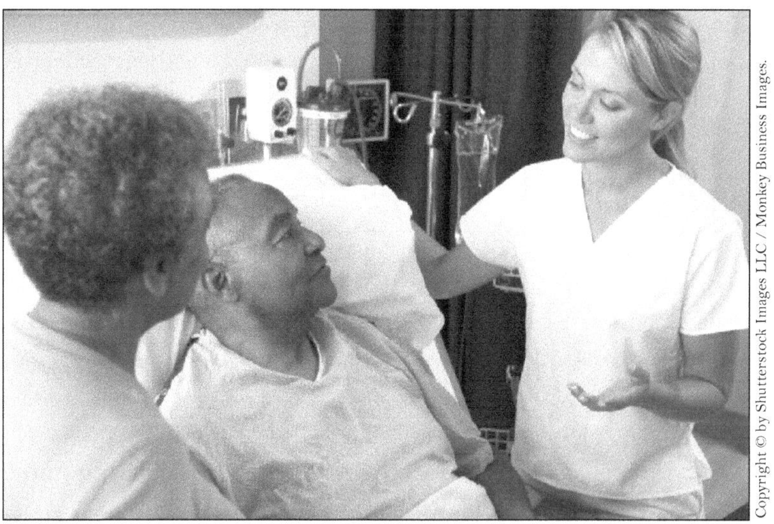

Clinical wisdom emerges as nurses increase in professional passion and knowledge. This passion and knowledge promote a transformation of understanding in nursing to clinical wisdom in the profession. This transition is immersed in the ethics and moral conduct that can be visualized as nursing excellence. As care becomes more complex and nursing knowledge, skills, and responsibilities increase, nurses will need to expand in acquisition and use of knowledge. These will promote management of current and potential patient problems in judgment decisions. This forethought will improve patient safety. The nurse will not just be involved, but engaged in care decisions, using ethics and clinical reasoning.

Clinical wisdom may be a standard expectation in practice. This form of thinking is mixed with theories and models in nursing to promote use of clinical wisdom to apply evidence-based interventions for patient health care outcomes. Benner et al. (1999) based clinical wisdom on clinical judgment and a thinking-in-action approach that incorporated feelings, emotions, and senses. They also identified thinking in action as a mechanism related to proficient nursing and expertise in the profession. In a study by Uhrenfeldt and Hall (2007), findings of participants in clinical practice identified that the most important elements to clinical practice were "the ability to think critically and with ethical discernment, and to act and practice responsibility by applying abstract thinking and knowledge to specific acts of care; that is, the proficient nurses showed clinical wisdom" (p. 391). The three themes that emerged from this research on clinical wisdom was to think, to act, and to be responsible. Proficient practice will consist of clinical wisdom based on these three themes.

In 2011 Benner, Kyriakidis, and Stannard published *Clinical Wisdom and Interventions in Acute and Critical Care: A Thinking-in-Action Approach.* In this document, they promote emphasizing learning *about* nursing rather than how to be a nurse. This thought is a challenge to education that will be engaged by programs as curriculum revisions occur. Activities that promote clinical experiences that result in the production of active thinking are already being used in educational programs through interactive clinical simulations. This mode of education will increase in frequency and acceptance for clinical educational experience. Nurse graduates will be able to actively reflect and effectively integrate information from classroom to clinical and from clinical to the classroom.

Nursing's Future Role

The pace of change is relentless and this will continue into the future. Society will maintain the need for the services of nurses, and their demand will be even greater as the future progresses. Nurses are the largest group of health care providers, and their needed numbers will continue to increase. The role of the nurse will continue to expand and the role of patient advocate will include more patient education and validation of compliance with health regimens. It is possible the nurse role will be more consultative rather than involve actual delivery (see Figure 2).

Nurses will use their knowledge base to be a professional patient partner and consultant for health care delivery. Self-care will be promoted through genomics

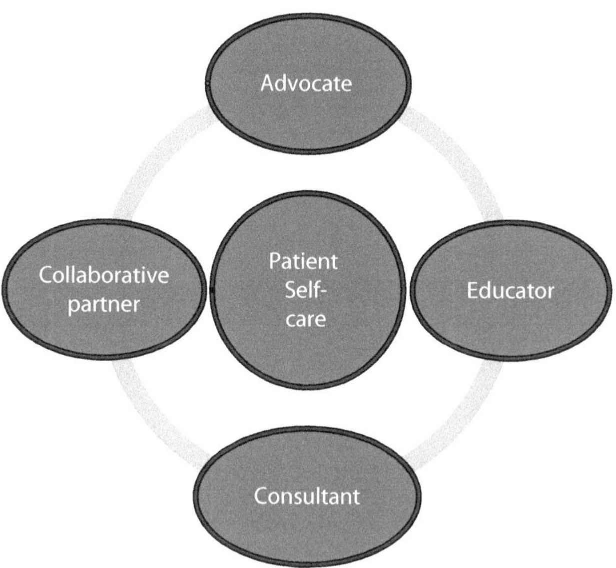

Figure 2. Nurse Role in Patient Partnership

and nanotechnological innovations. Patients will have astute knowledge of potential diseases that they self-monitor and use holistic mechanisms (nutritional, spiritual, pharmaceutical, psychological, and physiological) of care to manage. Nurses will continue to be primary information managers. They will collect data, transform this data into information for patient management, collaborate to integrate information from individual care providers and other records, analyze information, make decisions based on the data collected from technological and nontechnological means (nursing wisdom components), and effectively communicate this information to professional (other nurses, physicians, therapists, etc.) and nonprofessional (patient and family) care providers.

Health records will be open and readily accessible to patients. Individuals may be able to access their health record from any computer terminal. Health records will be seamless and interactive from any health delivery site. Nursing information placed on individualized records will be available for immediate review by the patient or any other health care provider with a need to know. Nurses will be more involved in politics and function in more collaborative health care organizational roles. Nursing will be dynamic in how it works in organizations. Research will be an expectation, and evidence-based practice will be the norm.

References

Barkan, S. Sociology: (2010). Understanding and changing the social world. Retrieved from http://www.flatworldknowledge.com/node/364134#web-364134

Benner, P., Hooper-Kyriakidis, P., & Stannard, D. (1999). *Clinical Wisdom and Interventions in Critical Care. A Thinking-in-Action Approach.* Saunders.

Benner, P., Kyriakidis, P., & Stannard, D. (2011). *Clinical Wisdom and Interventions in Acute and Critical Care.* New York: Springer Publishing.

Centers for Disease Control. Healthy People 2020. Retrieved from http://www.cdc.gov/nchs/healthy_people/hp2020.htm

Centers for Medicare and Medicaid Services, Office of the Actuary, National Health Statistics Group, National Health Care Expenditures Data, January 2010.

HealthCare.gov. The Health Care Law and You. Retrieved from http://www.healthcare.gov/law/introduction/index.html

Janzen, K. (2010). Alice Through the Looking Glass: The Influence of Self and Student Understanding on Role Actualization Among Novice Clinical Nurse Educators. *Journal of Continuing Education in Nursing,* 41(11), 517–523. doi:10.3928/00220124-20100701-07.

Millholland, K. (2001). *The Nursing Risk Management Series.* American Nurses Association. Retrieved from http://www.nursingworld.org/mods/archive/mod311/cerm201.htm

Nagle, L., & Yetman, L. (2009). Moving to a culture of nurse as knowledge worker and a new way of knowing in nursing. *Studies in Health Technology and Informatics,* 146467–472.

Paton, B. (2007). Knowing within: Practice wisdom of clinical nurse educators. *Journal of Nursing Education,* 46(11), 488–495.

Uhrenfeldt, L., & Hall, E. (2007). Clinical wisdom among proficient nurses. *Nursing Ethics,* 14(3), 387–398. doi: 10.1177/0969733007075886.

Villeneuve, M., & MacDonald, J. (2006). *Toward 2020: Visions for Nursing.* Ottawa, ON: Canadian Nurses Association. New York: Springer Publishing.

Index

Printed by Libri Plureos GmbH in Hamburg,
Germany